"No one knows their way around a candle [...] has been synonymous with candle magic [...] *Big Book of Candle Magic*, Jacki shares ever[...] preparing, using, and empowering candles to illuminate your life and bring big magic into all your endeavors. This extremely comprehensive guide, brimming with techniques and tips, is sure to level up your craft through the experience and expertise of someone who has devoted their life to the art of candles and their magic."

—Mat Auryn, author of *Psychic Witch*

"Candle magic is so much more than just a wick and a prayer. In this meaty tome, the irrepressible Jacki Smith offers us nothing less than her vast experience with making, dressing, and casting spells with candles, all within a friendly setting that is as approachable as it is full of wisdom. Let "Aunt Jacki" be your guide to making magic in your life. A masterclass on candle spells, this book has everything from the core basics to advanced techniques and everything in-between to take your spellcasting to the next level. Correspondences, types of candles, symbolism, journaling, divination, safety concerns, and even simply asking the right questions before you cast that spell, *The Big Book of Candle Magic* has everything you need to make your spells deeper and more effective. If you are wanting to learn more about magic and candle spells, in particular, then this book is for you."

—Storm Faerywolf, author of *The Witch's Name*

"At last! Jacki Smith—a woman who definitely knows her stuff when it comes to candle magic—has finally given us the gift for which we've all been waiting: a book not only filled with expert advice but also easy-to-apply tips and tricks to ensure that every candle spell hits its mark. *The Big Book of Candle Magic* should have a permanent home in every magical workspace, as it's a manual to which both beginners and seasoned practitioners will find themselves referring again and again."

—Dorothy Morrison, author of *Utterly Wicked*

"I love a book by Jacki Smith and *The Big Book of Candle Magic* is no exception. It is filled to the brim with Jacki's down-to-earth wisdom and experience, and you'll find so much to add to your candle-magic practice and you will thoroughly enjoy her unique take on spell casting."

—Madame Pamita, author of *The Book of Candle Magic*

"Jacki Smith delivers fresh and thorough insight into the subject of candle magic. Many of us have long relied on her well-crafted candles to support our magic, and this book is full of inspiration for new ways to ignite those flames. In this practical how-to book, Aunt Jacki encourages her readers to deepen their understanding of magic, along with their own motivations and true goals. Her voice is both educational and motivational, making *The Big Book of Candle Magic* a pleasure to read."

—Chas Bogan, author of *The Secret Keys of Conjure*

"Candle magic is an easy yet potent tool to incorporate into your spiritual practice. To learn the secrets to spell crafting and how to set your intentions, buy this illuminating book. Jacki Smith lights the way with sacred play!"

—Amy Zerner and Monte Farber, authors of *The Enchanted Tarot*

"Jacki Smith's direct, practical, matter-of-fact approach to magic makes it easily accessible to all. In *The Big Book of Candle Magic,* she invites you to take control of your power to manifest and direct it for very real results. Jacki has the wisdom, the tools, and the experience to validate her words, which you can rely on to pull you out of the sometimes difficult, sometimes conflicting, sometimes vague directions you might find in other magical texts. With ease and humor, Jacki gives you exactly what you need to navigate your dreams and make them a reality!"

—Susan Diamond, owner/operator of Moonstone Metaphysical
in Los Gatos, and Serpent's Kiss Magical and Crossroads
Community Space in Santa Cruz

"Over the years I've owned two occult stores, and I would have been overjoyed to have had *The Big Book of Candle Magic* by Jacki Smith on my shelves. It elegantly describes the how, when, and why of candles as a powerful focus and anchor for spells that address real world needs. It also manages to teach quite a bit about inner workings of magic without bogging down the flow of the practical material. Jacki Smith puts her life wisdom and positive outlook on almost every page. In addition to being a book about using candles for workings, it also offers suggestions on how to view yourself and how you make your way through the world. This broader perspective and clarity do as much to improve your spells as the excellent techniques that she shares. I will be buying it for myself and gifting it to others."

—Ivo Dominguez Jr., author of *Four Elements of the Wise*

"Have you been looking for a way to take your magic to the next level? Jacki Smith offers up a fresh perspective on candle magic, and it is an impressive one. Smart, savvy, and packed full of solid practical information, *The Big Book of Candle Magic* is a must-have for the modern practitioner."

—Ellen Dugan, author of *Garden Witchery*

"Jacki Smith has done it again! In her latest work, *The Big Book of Candle Magic*, she successfully marries magic with psychology. This book is not only a great read, but thoughtfully written, insightful, and transformative. Smith is truly an alchemist of the soul."

—Storm Cestavani, cohost of *Keep It Magic*

"*The Big Book of Candle Magic* is a fantastic, comprehensive guide and reference for budding and experienced magic-makers alike. Jacki shares sage wisdom for spellcasting that is steeped in spiritual integrity ensuring that the reader avoids pitfalls and heads straight into the gold of making high-vibrational magic. I'll be referring to this book to expand my own magic for years to come."

—Kerri Hummingbird, author of *The Second Wave*

"In the middle of this book is a cartoon of what we think magic should look like vs. what it actually looks like. It was funny, sharp, and insightful. So is the entire book. I grew up on candle magic books that told you the shape, color, oil, and prayers to use. Those are still great, but what Jacki does in this book is take you by the hand and walk you through the how and why of every aspect of this type of magic. From establishing the *why* that drives your spell, to the hidden principles behind the *how* and *what*, this book is a gift to anyone that cares about digging deeper than the recipe books."

—Jason Miller, author of *Consorting with Spirits*

THE BIG BOOK OF
CANDLE
MAGIC

JACKI SMITH

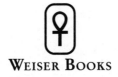

WEISER BOOKS

This edition first published in 2022 by Weiser Books, an imprint of

Red Wheel/Weiser, LLC
With offices at:
65 Parker Street, Suite 7
Newburyport, MA 01950
www.redwheelweiser.com

ISBN: 978-1-57863-763-8
Library of Congress Cataloging-in-Publication Data available upon request.

Cover design by Kathryn Sky-Peck
Cover photograph by Jacki Smith
Interior photographs by Jacki Smith
Interior illustrations by Dave Linabury, ArtOfDavezilla.com
Interior design by Debby Dutton
Typeset in Adobe Garamond, Frutiger LT, and Trajan Pro

Printed in Canada
MAR

10 9 8 7 6 5 4 3 2 1

This is a celebration of the past thirty years. Thirty years of making magical candles at Coventry Creations and thirty years of riding the business rollercoaster with my magical partner, Patty Shaw. Together, Patty and I have learned a lifetime of candle magic—inside and out. And, if given the chance, I would do it all over again with her every time.

There have also been a whole host of candlemakers or, as I like to call them, magic makers, over the past thirty years that deserve praise, appreciation, and dedication in this book. I can't name them all, but every employee of Coventry has left their mark, not only on our legacy but also on the world through the more than two million candles that we have made and sold. Every year I say, "This is the best team we have ever had!" We grow, evolve, and become even more magical over time. This year's team kept everything running while I focused on *The Big Book of Candle Magic;* they are the best team ever! Also, I'd like to give a special thanks to Storm Cestavani for being a part of this team and digging in deep with me.

Finally, this book could not have been written without the assistance of Rebecca Phoenix. She is my hero, and I am humbled that I get to be her mother. AG Phoenix gets the rest of this dedication as he provided my writing oasis, my bourbon, my balance, and my unwavering support system while simultaneously kicking my arse. Cheers.

CONTENTS

THE MAGIC
HOUR IS NOW

S o you want to do a candle spell? I like to start with the question, do you really need a spell?

But before we answer that, let's get on the same page and define what a *spell* is. My 21st-century interpretation of a spell is "a shifting of energy toward an intended goal." I see magic and spellwork all around us—in goal setting, emotional healing, self-care work, romancing, chanting, working out, as well as setting lights, ritual, ceremonies, charms, spells, and laying tricks. Wherever we focus our intent is magic.

A good spell has thoughtful ingredients and focused words of power and achieves the goal you want. The Joy of Spellcrafting and beyond of the *Big Book of Candle Magic* help you put the pieces together to create a *good* spell. A *great* spell addresses your whole life, how you react to your needs, what is broken and ready for healing, and how to create deep life changes with a series of candle spells. If you do the work, the Magic Hour Is Now section of the book will help you create a great spell.

This is the longest section of the *Big Book of Candle Magic* and many of you will skip it to jump into crafting your own spell. Once you have done that, come on back and go through these first exercises to unlock the magical secrets you have been keeping from yourself. This first part contains the big magic.

And to get into big magic, start with the question, "Do I need a spell?"

Probably.

If there is an issue that needs resolution, a well-directed candle spell will help. The impact of that spell depends on the prep work, your intention, and your commitment to a shift in energy. Magic begins and ends with your energy as it is—first and foremost, it's an internal process. With your spell you are altering *your* energy to create a change in your wider world. You begin with your need and end with the inner personal evolution that aligns with your intent. If you never shift your own energy to vibrate with this new idea you are creating, your success will be stalled or fleeting. If you are burning a candle to bring love into your life but you never heal the wound that keeps you feeling unloved, your magic will eventually feel unsuccessful.

Magic at its core is healing. When you embrace it in this way, you are working through the layers of wounds that limit your power and evolution.

Magic = healing

Healing = change

Change = magic

Do you need a spell? If you are ready to manifest a change and heal a need both in yourself and in the wider world, then *yes!*

Once you make your decision to step into a magical solution, it's time to get clear on what you are really asking for before you build that candle spell. The magic hour to create healing change in your life is *now*.

WHY CANDLE MAGIC?

The Law of Attraction (LoA) continues to be a growing movement. It's amazing how many seemingly mundane people I meet are invested in the Law of Attraction. It is wild to me that the idea of manifesting your dreams and wishes by focusing on energy is now the norm in so many non-magical circles.

Witches and magical practitioners know all about the Law of Attraction, since this is what many of us have been doing all along. What's the difference between LoA and magic? Tools.

In the words of witchcraft author Orion Foxwood, "Tools work when you can't." When you add the ritual of magic to your intent, even when you can't fathom how to manifest what you want, your intent will manifest faster and cleaner. And that is

Tip from your Aunt Jacki: If you want to see magic in action, sit in a room of entrepreneurs brainstorming new solutions to a problem. It's transformational.

where candle magic comes in. Candles provide an easy, powerful ritual within themselves. They are tools that transcend your current limitations. The physical process of burning a candle reflects the energetic transformation you experience during magic. When the energetic and the physical are aligned, they become a unified symbology that your emotional mind connects to, thus powering your magic up to the next level.

Candles are alchemy—they combine the five elements of the universe to create a new substance and transformation. Candles are themselves a perfect balance of the elements that together create the transformation. Let's take this apart:

Candles are made up of some type of wax, which comes from the earth in one way or another.

The wax must be heated to become liquid to mold it into a usable form: a process of fire and water.

Scent brings in the element of air.

You must have a wick—earth again.

The molten wax cools to become a usable candle—air.

You light the candle with fire.

The candle melts into molten wax—water.

The wax is pulled up the wick to feed the flame—earth and fire.

The wax is converted into a gaseous form—air.

The smoke rides up on the warm currents while transforming your intent into magic—air and spirit.

Your intent thus travels through every element, transforming over and over until it vibrates perfectly to manifest itself.

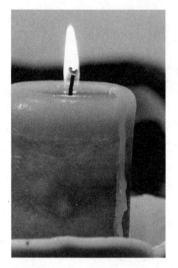

Every time a candle pees, a witch has cast her spell.

The flame of the candle is where heaven and earth meet. This beautiful sentiment reminds me that whenever we add magic into our lives, we are cocreating with the divine. The quickening of the flame brings divine influence closer and closer to you, helping you heal, manifest, transform, let go, and open up to what it will take to bring your spell into existence. When heaven and earth meet, magic is afoot.

DO YOU NEED A SPELL OR A REALITY CHECK?

The biggest barrier to getting what you want is "shoulding" on yourself. When you step out of what you think you *should* do, you step into the journey of finding out what you *really want*. If you know exactly what you want, most spells are pretty straightforward, and setting your intent will be a breeze. If you are already seeing your needs without a veil of society's expectations, skip ahead and scan the sample spells on page 181 to get started on crafting your own candle spell. But if you are not so sure about what you want or are stuck on what you *should* do, stay with me here, and I will show you how to get a crystal clear picture of what your desires really are so you can cast your intent and direct your spells.

Crafting a spell is like reading the instructions on the side of a microwave meal. There is no tone, inflection, or emotional urgency in a spell; there are only literal directions. I love telling a cautionary tale of doing money spells and how I was kind of bad at it in the beginning. In my initial spells, I smartly set the intent for more money in my life. Psychics were telling me that money surrounded me, yet my financial issues were not resolving. Then I woke up to the fact that I was surrounded by people doing well financially. My inner circle, surrounding me, *were* chock-full of money, and yet I was not doing as well as them. Huh. Missed that one by an inch, and I missed it by a mile.

Round 2: I clarified my intent to increase the money coming to *me*. Then my bills went up. Yes, more money was flowing to me and then flowing right out again. Everything that needed fixing and replacing started making itself known, and I was cash poor once again.

Round 3: I got even smarter and stepped into the literal directions of my intent. I declared that my revenue and profits would grow. Bingo! It happened: my revenue grew; my profits grew and found stability for a time. Unfortunately, *I* didn't grow. Instead, I rested on my success. This lack of an energetic shift within me made my spellwork fleeting, and I crashed hard, again.

I can apply this scenario to any magical subject—relationships, protection, healing, clearing. Our magical intent works on the level where we currently reside. When we find success and level up, our intent needs to level up too. This is one of the wonders of spiritual development: it's never boring, and there is forever a new epiphany right around the corner, making your intention work an evolving practice. We forget that what we really want evolves with us. Every year I update my life and business goals, so why not my intentions too? And over that time my intention setting has evolved into "I am safe and secure in my finances, and I have a clear understanding and wisdom of how to make them grow in a sustainable way."

Humor me and set aside your intention-setting expertise. Now do this exercise with me:

Grab your Candle Magic Journal. (You have a journal ready for the work, don't you? Not quite? Go get one. I'll wait.) Then write down answers to the following questions:

> What are you struggling with or where do you feel limited right now?

Tip from your Aunt Jacki: Doing these exercises might seem awkward and tedious at first and you will want to skip to the end. Stick with me at least once before you jump. After you practice a couple of times, setting your intent from a deeper level will become second nature. Then, eventually, something else will be the new and shiny magical idea and you will forget all about this process. We all need to revisit the basics now and then, and it's a good thing to have these directions when you need them. How do I know this is how things go? I do it too.

What are you feeling right now?

What do you want to be feeling right now?

What support, wisdom, or resources do you have right now?

What support, wisdom, or resources are you open to receiving?

Finally, make a statement of how your life is now that you have resolved the issue at hand and received the resources you're open to. State this as if it has already happened and end it with, "That or something even better."

You've just created the basis for your intent and the words of power for your spell, along with a growth clause. Save this. We are going to look at it again when it's time to hone your words of power.

SHE WHO ASKS THE QUESTIONS . . . IS IN CONTROL OF THE OUTCOME

She who asks the questions, rules the room.

—Jacki Smith

Have you ever noticed that the person in the room who asks the questions is in charge of the conversation? They direct the attention where they want it to go. They drive the narrative and can actually control the response. It may seem like the person answering is in charge, but look closer and you'll see they are responding, not directing.

I became aware of this every time I took an entrepreneurial class or started to engage a coach. I came into the room with what I wanted to get out of the situation and ended up realizing I needed something else. Watch a good salesperson at work and you'll see that they ask questions and do less of the talking until the end. Teachers do this as well to engage their students. Leaders do this to understand their team and eventually funnel their energy in the direction needed. This technique creates alignment, engagement, and belief.

Magically speaking, if you ask yourself deep-diving questions about your spell, you get your mind, emotions, spirit, and even body engaged in the same way in the success of your spell. You begin to believe in your ability to shift your energy and make magic happen.

CANDLE MAGIC JOURNALING

This book is a guide to understanding how candle magic can work for you. I am pulling together more than three decades of experience in a way that can be easily referenced so you can experiment with your own candle magic practice. There is a bookshelf in my office that houses thirty years of notes on candles, magic, healing, and more. I will randomly pick up a notebook, flip it open, and remember where I was at that point of my life and what my magic taught me. I am the only one who fully understands my notes, because I have the memory of what got me there. It is the backstory that makes the magical conclusion so powerful. You are starting your own journey now, so start your own Candle Magic Journal. Not every color, ingredient, or recommended wording will work for you. But if you track your choices and magical progress, you can, most possibly, avoid doing the same thing over and over again that is not giving you the results you are looking for.

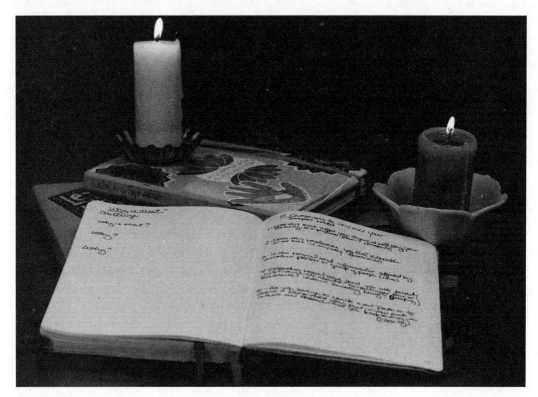

Candle magic journaling—your future self will thank you.

I understand the habit of hoarding lovely leather-bound journals and precious blank books with gorgeous art and precious inner pages with icons and art. For years, I didn't write a bit in any of the fine journals I owned. I finally became a successful journal keeper when I picked up the 99-cent back-to-school reject in the clearance bin. This was disposable. I didn't have to be perfect with my penmanship, thoughts, and words. I was able to stream consciousness—or insanity as it were—onto the pages and come to a place where I understood my deeper need. So grab some cheap notebooks and follow me into crafting your own magical candle practice.

Oh, and if you need an idea of what to jot down, there are lots of exercises in this chapter that require paper and pen. At the very least, put down what you are doing. The candle, the intent, the words of power, the day, date, and time, and anything else you add to the spell. Jot down how the candle is burning, what is happening in your day-to-day, and how long it took for you to start seeing small energetic shifts in your life. The more you practice this, the better you get at it, but if you are like me, your journaling will be inconsistent at best. Don't sweat it—my thirty years of inconsistent journaling has still become a treasure trove of information today.

Tip from your Aunt Jacki: If you want to set your Candle Magic Journal up for more organized tracking of your spellwork, follow the journaling prompts throughout this book and you will become a pro in no time at all. You don't have to be *perfect*, you just have to begin. Make it, make it good, then make it better. That is how we master a thing.

THE DEEPER NEED

In the 21st century, many of us are forced to live our lives in a high-octane environment. Go fast and burn out. Deal with the crisis of the day; respond and react to a stimulus and then move on to the next one. There is an overwhelming amount of input to process every day, and often we lose track of our own inner voice amid the louder voices coming through the media, social and otherwise. We have input in nearly every moment of our lives directing our responses and fighting for our attention. Eventually, our inner world fills with this cacophony of mental noise and we stop processing what is happening around and to us.

Magically, as we start to respond to the external physical environment only, our spells become shallow quick fixes. These surface-level spells are bandages for the deeper wound and the deeper need and will eventually feel like they fail. I know you want to settle your issue right now, stop the pain, resolve the emergency. No one likes to sit in discomfort. Work with me for a few moments before you light that revenge candle to understand your true deeper need. Slow down and allow your spirit and inner voice to clear out the noise and catch up to you through the pain. You have a deeper need that you have been hiding from yourself. Approaching your magic from this slower pace can create a life-changing result or, at the minimum, be more effective. It's OK to be in pain and discomfort for a moment as this holds the wisdom you need to find the root of the problem.

Nothing in your life happens in a vacuum. Your needs for money, companionship, protection, peace, and other things did not appear spontaneously. Every need comes from a collection of experiences and decisions, by you and others, that culminated in the current emergency. When you can track the path that caused your emergency or discomfort, you shift yourself from victimhood to personal power. The passive becomes the active. Whether by your own hand or those of others, you have more power than the momentum of the crisis. Accepting a passive identity in victimhood robs you of your ability to actively correct and work against these negative situations. An emergency is an act done against us, not an identity we are required to accept.

HOW WE TRICK OURSELVES—THE POWER OF SELF-IDENTIFICATION

No one wants to be the bad guy in their own story. We have lots of reasons why we can't, don't, are not destined to, or are terminally misunderstood. This is how we trick ourselves into letting go of our power and embracing the victimization of our world. We are masters at this and learned from the best—our ego. The job of the ego is to protect us from pain and fear, to keep us from destroying our sense of self and losing our identity. It does this by creating beliefs that hold us in our uncomfortable comfort of being the hero in a world of villains. We trick ourselves into staying stagnant and in line with the status quo. If the status quo worked as well as our ego is telling us it does, we wouldn't be looking for a magical solution for the challenges in front of us.

Tip from your Aunt Jacki: It's not victim-blaming to understand your part in the story. Getting clarity on your own actions and thought forms pulls your energy back to you and allows you to trust yourself again. Let go of any self-blame and look at the experience as something that is not required to hold power over you.

I love the ego. When it is healthy, it saves you in times of trauma, helps you create boundaries, and assists you in finding your sense of purpose. If you challenge yourself, your ego, to embrace where you could have been the villain in your own story, you awaken a healthy shadow side of your magic that will help you grow. Shadows are not bad or evil; they are the place where we can relax from the onslaught of too much input and find our truth. Remember, we don't grow in the light; that's where we collect our food or information. We grow in the shadows where we can process that food or information and use it to evolve. Step into the shadows with me and find your deeper magical need, your "why" for casting your spell.

By stepping into the shadows you will be letting go of your logical brain and listening to your primal instincts and intuition. Your instincts speak fast and creatively. Do not try to interpret them at the moment, because that is where you will trick yourself. When my instincts go off, I flow into them. I ask if this is a fear, block, belief, or lie that I tell myself. I flow deeply into it at the moment and let it give me all the information it has. There may be no logical answer to anchor this instinct to, so if the intuition is way out there, I will watch and wait.

In the fall of 2019, my instincts were screaming that my company Coventry needed to overstock all of our products. I saw that sales were steadily growing, but the level of overstock that my primal brain was pushing me toward was well beyond the sales projections. I wondered if January was going to be particularly busy. As a team, we supported my instincts and decided to stock our candles and raw materials deeper than we ever had before. January of 2020 was a high sales month, and yet, I kept us at a higher stock level of candles and raw materials. Then the pandemic hit. This high level of inventory and raw material that my intuition kept telling me to create kept us in business during the shutdown. Shipping was disrupted in a way the 21st century had never seen before. If we hadn't had that product waiting, we would not have survived. My instincts also told me to close down a few days before the state mandated it. I didn't know then that I had contracted COVID-19 and was about to be highly contagious. The following four weeks were the sickest I had ever been in my life, and since there were no tests available, the doctors kept telling me it was a horrible flu. A June 2020 antibody test confirmed that I indeed had COVID-19, and, thankfully, I hadn't spread it to anyone else in my company. This was all a result of a developed intuition that I have been honing for thirty years.

Your primal instincts have the key to your deeper need—your why—and yet we trick ourselves into discounting them because they are not logical enough. Put away your logic and play with finding your why.

GETTING IN TOUCH WITH YOUR WHY

My book *Coventry Magic* was published in 2011, before I ever heard of Simon Sinek and his best-selling book *Start with Why.* In *Coventry Magic* I have a chapter called And I Cry, "Why?!" where I share how to evaluate your deeper magical need and cast a spell that addresses that need. It's a cornerstone of *Coventry Magic* and a powerful tool that I not only use daily, but also teach in every class. Getting in touch with the deeper why of any situation is the empowerment that can skyrocket your spell. Imagine my excitement, two years after writing this book, in coming across Sinek's TED Talk and subsequently his book where he introduced the Golden Circle that leaders use to find the why of their business. Sinek shows in his Golden Circle that there are three layers to any business or product: the *what* (the product), the *how* (the process or what it does), and the often missed *why* (the reason you are in business). If you build your business on the *what* or the *how*, you are less likely to create a sustainable business that inspires loyalty. If you build your business on the *why*, you inspire your customers and staff to invest their emotions and subsequent loyalty into your product and brand. I love a good universal synchronicity and feel deep in my core that entrepreneurship is magic for the business world. We all need our core why to empower and inspire us.

For instance: I could cast a spell for protection, but if I don't understand my deeper need, my why, I could totally miss the mark. Missing the mark might mean an unsuccessful spell, or it might be that my friends stop calling because they don't feel connected to me anymore. It might be that I really don't believe in my power to cast an effective spell. It was just a candle that I lit, and it didn't work.

Whether in a business setting or a magical setting, we naturally start with the logical brain and what we need. I logically need to increase my income because my rent went up. I logically need to create more harmony in my home to bring peace to everyone. Logic goes only so far in inspiring energy, though, especially if you have no idea *how* you are going to get there. Yes, magic and intention setting are very literal and logical, but they need the emotional *why* to power them. Letting go of the logical *what* can be very scary because you are dropping yourself into the sea of unexplored emotions. Using the "Why Is That?" exercise allows you to dip your toe into the sea of emotions, gently walking to a depth you can handle today. Tomorrow, you may find the strength to go in a little deeper and eventually learn to swim.

The "Why Is That?" exercise allows you to hang on to the logical and safe *what* while uncovering your *how* and empowering it with your *why*. When all three are in play, you are in the Golden Circle of magic where you are empowered to support a transformation with candle magic that can be life-changing.

"Why Is That?" Exercise

1. Settle in, get comfy, get out paper and pen, and breathe.
   Fold your paper in thirds like a letter in an envelope, and then unfold it.
   Write your challenge, issue, or wish on the top of your paper.
   Directly under your challenge write, "Why is that?"
   Just below the first fold write, "Why?"

Just below the second fold write "Why?" one more time.
Refold your paper in thirds, with the issue on the top.

2. Close your eyes, and breathe in and out three times in the biggest way
you can. Throw some drama into it because you are letting go of the
tension of the day. Lift your shoulders on
the inhale and drop them on the exhale.
Your next three breaths will be slow, calm,
and easy. Relax into your thoughts and let
them unwind into what you are challenged
with. Let yourself fall into it, with all of
your frustrations, fears, worries, and needs.
Get a little worked up.

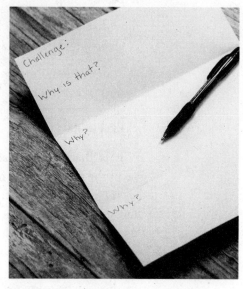

NOW! Look at your paper and the
question, "Why is that?" Write down the
immediate thing that comes to mind. This
is the reaction you have in the nanosecond
of asking why. You want the immediate
primal response to your question. It won't
make sense. It may be weird random
words. Actually, if it's not weird random
words, start again. Go back into your
relaxed state and feel your problem from

Write it down to limit your self-delusion.

head to toe, get stressed and emotional, and then ask, "Why is that?"
Write down what your primal instincts want to tell you and flip your
folded paper to the next "Why?"

3. Relax again into your first answer that does not make sense. Think
about it in all directions, mull over how it connects to your issue. Feel
confused if needed, get angry, frustrated, let your emotions roll.

NOW! Let your eyes fall on the question, "Why?" and let the
primal brain respond in a nanosecond again and write down what pops
into your head.

4. Turn the paper to the next "Why?" and start to drift into these answers.
Allow a thread to move from these words to the first set of words to
your issue. Let your thoughts spin a little with confusion, inspiration, or
any other experience you are having. Float into your last set of answers
and then . . .

NOW! Look at your paper and answer the third "Why?" This series of answers will start to make more sense. Jot down the words quickly, allowing your primal instincts to get to the core of what is bothering you. If you feel there is more, add another "Why?" to the back of your paper and go for round four. It's OK, I often have to go four levels deep before I stop.

5. Unfold your paper and underline or circle the words that feel like they are telling the tale of what your deeper need is.

6. Your end result may look nothing like where you started, and that is normal and expected. It's OK, you are tuning in to your primal instinct to guide you on what magic you really need to make the bigger change in your life.

"Why Is That?" works best with two people: one guide, one responder. The goal of the guide is to get the responder into the alpha state of meditation so they can pull up all the discomfort of the challenge and then startle them into allowing the primal instincts to speak. Really, it is different every time. When I do this in classes I teach, my students become very emotionally vulnerable with their answers, and I honor them by being nonreactive and mindful of how this may affect them. When you choose a partner to do this with, make sure they can be trusted with the vulnerability you will open up to.

I once had an individual become distraught when I took her through the "Why Is That?" exercise. She was not expecting this and didn't have time to rationalize her answers. This allowed us to reveal some deep energetic wounds that she was then empowered to address. She surprised herself, as her deeper need went from a money spell into healing her relationship with her father who had always told her she was not enough. (The healing was with her energetic relationship as she had cut ties with her father.)

Sometimes the why has no clear answer, and you need to trust yourself when that happens. Remember my story about stocking my candles deep? I did the "Why Is That?" exercise several times. The final answer kept coming back, "You will need it." It went something like this:

Challenge: I can't shake the panicked feeling that we need to double stock. We don't have this much money to risk on this.

Why is that? *You don't have enough stock right now.* (Though, we had our standard three weeks' worth of product.)

WHY is that not enough? *You will need it.*

WHY will I need this product? *YOU WILL NEED IT!*

Got it. We will need it.

I also use this when I am freaking out to start to calm myself down.

Challenge: I am emotionally destroyed by an argument I had with my husband. I just want to run away from the horrid pain. I am going to leave.

Why is that? *I am so scared of his response.*

Why? *What if this is a permanent rift?*

Why? *I am terrified he won't love me, and I love him so much.*

I was able to calm down and get to my real fear. In this instance, I went back with a bit more clarity and started the conversation with, "I love you and I want us to work through this together. Do you want the same?" Game changer.

This process can also seem embarrassing. I once had a student publicly challenge me to the point of embarrassment, but I stuck with the process and we got a huge breakthrough. I asked for a volunteer who had a spell in mind that they wanted to cast. The most challenging, obstinate person in the class raised their hand lightning fast. Here is how it went:

Me: Think about your challenge or issue and the spell you want to do. Let it roll around in your head and really get into the emotions of the problem. Feel this problem in your head, heart, spirit, and body. Even get a little tense about it. When I ask you the next question, answer with the first thing that pops into your head. Just blurt it out. (—PAUSE—)

WHY IS THAT?

Student: *I want to f*ck (insert name) in my group.*

Me: (Thinking, "Oh crap, what do I do with this jerk!?") WHY IS THAT?

Student: *She is lonely and feels terrible about herself, and I want to show her she is beautiful.*

Me: ("Oh crap" some more) WHY?

Student: *She is a beautiful person inside and out. She was abused by her ex and believes the lies he told her. I don't know how to help her.*

Me: OK—we got somewhere with this. (Whew!) Do you see what magic would be most helpful in this situation?

Student: *Yes, I need to do confidence spells and cleansing spells with her. I need to do communication spells for myself so I know how to talk to her.*

Me: (blink, blink) OMG—You got it! What about that first statement you made?

Student: *That's the first thing that popped into my head to make someone feel better.*

Me: So we avoided a tricky situation where you would have thrown love spells out and not helped the situation and possibly hurt her more.

"Why Is That?" can take you into weird and tricky places, but keep asking why until you get to an answer that really rings your bell as the deeper truth.

If you need more help with this exercise and a magical partner is not available, you can use an oracle that will give you keywords. Tarot works really well with the "Why Is That?" exercise if you use the accompanying booklet to pull out meanings. If you interpret the cards on your own, you can trick yourself into staying in the logic. You need standard definitions to become the oracle of your deeper consciousness.

I HAVE MY WHY—NOW WHAT DO I DO?

Here you are with these ideas of what you really need magical assistance on. You have uncovered lots of keywords, deep-diving emotions, and possibly some weirdness that makes no sense. How does this become the foundation of candle magic? Maybe it doesn't. Do you need a spell here? You are at a pivot point where you decide: "yes, I want to craft a bit of candle magic to propel me on my journey," or "no, I think I need to focus my magic on my daily activities and create magic this way."

For the purpose of this book, you are choosing "yes, I want to craft a bit of candle magic."

Congratulations! You are stepping into advanced candle magic. Basic candle magic is lighting a candle. The minute you add to your candle spell you have advanced to the head of the class. This is where your Candle Magic Journal is important for the exploration of creating, executing, and reviewing any candle spell you attempt. With the clarity of hindsight, you can see the progression of your spells. Magic can be a form of healing if you let it. I dare you to look at your candle spells as a path of personal and spiritual growth. Choosing to learn from your challenges turns them into blessings and transforms you from a victim to your own personal hero. In the end, the only person you can count on saving you is you.

Start this self-saving process by titling your page with your original spell idea. Example: "Make More Money," "Bring Peace into the House," "Get Him to Call Me." List the questions and answers that got you clear on your intent earlier in this chapter. Follow this up with your results from the "Why Is That?" exercise. Include every crazy, weird word and response. *Do not edit.* This is where your intuitive, primal, and magical self is talking to you. If you edit or apply logic here, you are shutting off the magical power it is bringing to you, so *don't judge!* You can, however, add to it if you are experiencing insight or emotions around what you are copying. Once you get it all down, take a moment. Walk away, make a cup of tea, stretch, flip the laundry, vacuum—essentially put your attention on some other part of your life that needs self-care. Avoid texting, calling, social media, TV, or anything that takes you out of focusing internally. Take a ten- to thirty-minute pause and come back to your Candle Magic Journal, rereading it start to finish, and look for a pattern.

Read it aloud to yourself and feel how that radically changes your connection to the words on that paper. When you read aloud, you are inviting your whole essence to listen. Even the softest voice takes these words out of your circular thoughts and helps you hear yourself, your truth. Imagine you are telling a trusted confidant what you wrote down and actually listen to yourself. If you didn't find a pattern before, you will pick one up now. Something will really stand out, and you will begin to understand how you want your intention to evolve.

Tip from your Aunt Jacki: Personally, I find that a bit of candle magic—the right candle magic—can enhance any situation. Even the most mundane issues, like cleaning the house, deserve to be extraspecial, so I will light a spiritual cleansing candle, a Happy Home candle, and maybe a prosperity candle to fill my space with blessings.

Write down the patterns you found, your reactions, and what you really want out of this spell. Be courageous and let yourself feel the bigger desire. That bigger desire is the magical rocket fuel that will make your spell wildly successful . . . or it is the underground saboteur that will make your spell crash and burn.

IT'S OK TO ASK FOR WHAT YOU WANT

Tip from your Aunt Jacki: It always goes a little differently in your head because your thoughts do not need to be based in any reality. Read or say aloud any circular or obsessive thoughts and you can stop them from influencing every decision and action.

It's normal to walk into the magical world afraid to ask for what you really want. As a child, you were taught how to govern the need for immediate gratification. To become a productive part of the community, you are taught to hold back, make room for others, temper your greed, and take turns. These lessons—along with don't run with scissors and wash your hands—are all a part of what it takes to be a compassionate and respected member of society. In magic, it's a little bit different . . . In magic, we search for the bigger, deeper desire and make room for it to become part of our reality. If we don't get in touch with what we *really* want, we can sabotage the spell we are creating. Tap into the childlike freedom to ask for what you truly desire.

I would like to call for a moratorium on the fear of casting a spell that is for your own benefit. I am declaring a cease and desist order on the idea that your magical win will cause someone else to lose. Your prosperity spell is not going to cause Great Uncle Joe to die. That's not how it works. It's more likely to help Great Uncle Joe's lawyer to find your contact information. Magic taps into Universal Abundance where there is always enough. When we ask for what we really want, we are aligning our magic with Universal Abundance and teaching ourselves on every level that there will be enough. Holding back and being afraid that you are greedy validate the belief that there will always be a lack. What we believe, we manifest.

If your bigger desire is not lining up with your spell, that bigger desire will cause enough energetic dissonance to sabotage your success. Think about it this way: Your neighbor is having a loud party while you are trying to watch TV. Your attention will be continually pulled to the noise outside of your home, and you'll miss half the program. Your bigger desire is to be at the neighbor's party, but you weren't invited. It will be an obnoxious distraction until you pay attention to it. We have to be courageous enough to knock on the door of what we really want and find out our invitation got lost in the mail. You are not alone if you can't believe that what you really want is possible. Most of us have to step into this gradually because we've buried what we desire so damn deep and, once we find it, it's in another language. If you keep aligning yourself with Universal Abundance, you will learn the language of what you really want and be able to manifest it.

> **Tip from your Aunt Jacki:** Greed is a state of mind that occurs when you believe there is not enough and you are deprived of what you feel is your fair share. Greed is a belief that can be healed through gratitude, the generosity of love, and connecting to the universal source of abundance.

WHY WE HOLD BACK

The bigger desire can be truly terrifying. What if your bigger desire is to have friends to travel with, yet your crew has neither the desire nor the money. That is scary. Does that mean you need different friends? Will your current tribe forsake you if you travel with others? Every new thing does bring an end to something else, yet we can't predict what the trade-off will be. Again, scary.

The one thing I can tell you is that people who are truly evolving and looking for the blessing within every challenge don't regret the trade-off. Most are actually relieved. Going for the dream is a risk, a big risk. What if you don't succeed? It's true that if you never try, you won't fail. It is also true that success comes only after trying. Then there is the fear of what you are going to do after you get what you want. Will you be a different person?

Magic demands change. Again, if there's no need for change, there's no need for magic. Candle magic is the easy part. Evolving to sustain the change that candle magic brings you is more difficult. There is nothing more enticing than our old, uncomfortable comfort zone. We know how to manage it, complain about it, and work around it. It's steady and predictable. Magical change is not.

> **Tip from your Aunt Jacki:** Success may not change you, but retaining that success does. To live a different life, you have to *be* different, and you don't know what that difference will be until you get there. Supporting yourself with candle magic helps, as does therapy. This is a great time to clear out the old beliefs that have kept you from reaching the success you desire.

IT ALL COMES DOWN TO THE MAGIC 5

One thing I've learned along the way in my thirty years of magical exploration is there are five branches of magic work: Prosperity (any material gain), Protection (safety, stability, and peace), Love (any relationship), Clearing (removing an external block), and Healing (any internal change). You may wonder how I got to this conclusion, and you may even think I am flat-out wrong. What about spirit work, creativity, psychic development, family, control and compel spells, communication, garden spells, and everything else? In 2006 when I created my first spiral-bound *Pick a Candle Guide*, I had ten sections in it. Tranquility, inspiration and creativity, inner growth, guidance and wisdom, and home and family were the extra sections in the flip chart where I explored the Coventry candles you could combine to fulfill your magical need. It was a rabbit hole. The more I divided and conquered the what-if scenarios, the less it fit the need of anyone reviewing the guide.

In 2011 when I accidentally created the Coventry Magic Oracle deck, I had limited space, and so I had to keep it concise. I limited myself to five branches of magical intent. Decades of psychic readings and magical consultations brought me to the philosophy that any need or questions fell into one of the Magic 5. My clients wanted to know when their ship was coming in, is their soul mate on it, will their love heal all of their issues, and will they get revenge on all the haters in their life. This happy oracle accident, like many others that have shaped my magical practice, and Jacki's Magic 5 theory became a deep understanding of how we can take the chaos of emotions and circumstances and funnel it into simpler and more powerful life-changing magic.

The response to the Coventry Magic Oracle and my Magic 5 theory led to many discussions on how every question fit the model. I had to prove my theory with the most important people in the magical world—the store owner—and I converted many. I invited more challenges to my Magic 5 theory, and my business partner (aka my sister), customers, colleagues, and other magical authors all tried to find something that did not fit.

But for spell after spell, issue after issue, reading after reading—everything has a place in the Magic 5. Why did this work so well? This Virgo takes nothing on spec. I had to *understand* how this worked so well, and then I remembered my Psych 101 and Maslow's hierarchy of needs.

MASLOW'S HIERARCHY OF MAGIC?

In 1943 Abraham Maslow (April 1, 1908–June 8, 1970) introduced the hierarchy of needs describing five levels of human needs that must be met to achieve self-actualization. If the need in the level below is not met, it is impossible to find fulfillment in the next level. This theory became a popular framework for modern sociology and psychology. You can also find this theory in management and leadership training—if your staff is not getting their base needs met, they are hard-pressed to be productive in their job.

According to Maslow, the hierarchy of needs are physiological, safety, love, esteem, and self-actualization. While I was challenging myself to prove the Magic 5, I easily saw the synchronization with Maslow's theory. It's hard to feel really spiritual when you are worried about money or safety. Light bulbs turned on and I understood why I keep coming back to the Magic 5 in all areas of my work, how I advise, and how I teach.

Tales from your Aunt Jacki: Early in the days of witchery for me, I was lamenting to one of my magical mentors that I didn't feel very elevated. I wasn't having the amazing spiritual experiences my other coven members were. My psychic abilities were getting spotty, and I was feeling terrible about myself. Kevin looked me square in the face and said, "It's hard to feel the divine when your belly is empty, your husband is scaring off your friends, and you are worried for your safety. Focus your magic here and the rest will follow. Now, go look up Maslow's hierarchy of needs and get your shit together." Kevin was the type of guy who would slip extra cash into my bag when he knew I was struggling and got me a few reading gigs to gain experience and some income. He is not confrontational at all, so I knew he really came out of pocket to push me. He changed my life with that statement, and I did go look up Maslow and keep this as part of my own magical framework.

The Magic 5 represent the deeper need or the deficit in your life that could use a power-up. In other words, when you need a spell, you are repairing a deficit in a base survival requirement. We are complex beings at our core, and attaining the desired success of your spell may mean you are working many areas of magic at the same time. The Magic 5 don't have hard boundaries between them, but instead blend between the levels just like Maslow's hierarchy. Diving deep in your why will get you to the most basic need in your spells, then rocket your magical results all the way to self-actualization in a heartbeat. The manifestation of the spell is in essence self-actualization, and this is achieved in moments of clarity. We can't stay static in self-actualizations because we are always throwing a new challenge at ourselves to grow and evolve from. We can't grow at the top of our game, so we must climb down from the mountain. Even the Fool's Journey of the tarot puts the wise Hermit that lives at the top of the mountain as a perfect completion at number nine, which is quickly followed by the Wheel of Fortune that can pull you right off the mountain.

Dive deep through the Magic 5 and the hierarchy of needs and visit the "Why Is That?" exercise one more time to see if the answers you uncovered are deep enough to propel your magic to the top of the mountain of success.

Prosperity Magic = Physiological Needs

These are the main requirements for human survival. These are universal needs of air, water, food, sleep, health, clothes, and shelter. Maslow says, "For the man who is extremely and dangerously hungry, no other interest exists but food. He dreams food, he remembers food, he thinks about food, he emotes only about food, he perceives only food and he wants only food."

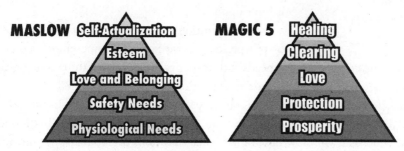

Maslow and magic—the synchronicity is divine.

This extreme need also defines what utopia looks like when one lives in this desperation: it is a place where these universal needs are met. "If only he were guaranteed food for the rest of his life, he would be perfectly happy and never want anything more. . . . Freedom, love, community feeling, respect, philosophy, may all be waved aside as fripperies, which are useless since they fail to fill his stomach."

Your base needs and how you define their minimum level are subjective, related to the time you live in, your social class, and your culture. It is rare for a person in today's modern industrialized nation community to experience the life-threatening hunger that is represented in the most basic aspect of physiological need. When the bar is raised to our middle-class view on survival, we redefine that physiological need to be the quality of life that we are living. That man who was starving and defined everything by food in Maslow's take becomes a man who is starving for something else in his life: love, esteem, health, validation, etc. When this hunger exists, the physiological needs are still triggered, bringing your magical need back to prosperity—in love, safety, companionship, etc. When this hunger exists, gratification and deprivation are equally motivating factors in your magic.

When you fill this need magically, you are able to move on to higher thinking through the next levels of needs. If your success is thwarted or deprived repeatedly, then you can't find the stability in this level, and your focus can't move from here. There are people whose needs in this area have always been satisfied, so when they face an unusual deficit, there is a belief that "of course, this will be solved as it has always been solved in the past." That belief goes a long way to empowering your magic—so long of a way that a whole philosophy of the Law of Attraction is built upon it.

Epiphany from your Aunt Jacki: The need for sexual fulfillment belongs in this level of Maslow's needs. It's not a companionship or love thing: it's a physiological need. No wonder so many of the ingredients for money double as attractants for a little lovin'.

Your definition of prosperity is not my definition of prosperity, yet we have the same emotional and energetic crisis when our needs for prosperity are not met. The physiological needs are very primal; they drive the actions of all furred, finned, and feathered creatures. Prosperity magic that taps into wild primal energy is powerful, yet fast and fleeting at the same time. It is hard to stay in this vibration all the time, as it will slow down the higher vibrations of hope, inspiration, and divine guidance.

Protection Magic = Safety Needs

Once there is food in your belly and a roof over your head—even metaphorically—you can start to be concerned about safety. War, natural disasters, economic disasters, abuse, or even job insecurity will derail your safety needs and create a desire for protection magic. Safety and protection are very pervasive in the core why of your spell. Maslow describes the broader aspects of safety needs as "the very common preference for familiar rather than unfamiliar things, or for the known rather than the unknown." I call this the uncomfortable comfort zone. Maslow further explains, "The tendency to have some religion or world-philosophy that organizes the universe and the men in it into some sort of satisfactorily coherent, meaningful whole is also in part motivated by safety seeking."

Aunt Jacki Theory #65: When the fear of the unknown is greater than the pain of staying where you are, you are in an uncomfortable comfort zone. It's time to pull up your big kid drawers and face that fear. It's usually just a little bugger that is making a big noise.

Safety needs of a personal nature, emotional vulnerability, financial security, and well-being all live in this level and are common themes in protection magic. This is typically a lonely place. When your safety is threatened, you can quickly retreat to feeling alone. Your own lens of pain is the only one you can see through, making you feel like you are the only one experiencing this trauma. Abuse can keep you stuck at this level, as the goal of any abuser or oppressor is to stay in control by keeping you isolated. This lack of safety can devolve into becoming the bully and attacker yourself. When you are abused and controlled, the backlash is to gain control over your own being in any way you can, including taking on that bully role. Stepping into that role keeps you isolated and prevents movement from this level.

Paranoia is born at this level and can keep you here by blocking your ability to discern what is dangerous and what is a manufactured response to continual fight-or-flight responses. Magic is driven by the state of our psyche, and one that is stressed will make reactionary choices. Paranoia and a constant feeling of impending doom are an extreme example of a deficit in your safety. A deficit can also show itself in subtler ways, like how we communicate with the people around us, feeling aggressive, or even attacking before we are attacked. Quick, aggressive responses to any attack at all are a symptom of a safety/protection need.

When your prosperity/physiological and protection/safety needs are managed and in balance, love, family, and companionship magic will become easier. As Maslow said, "He will hunger for affectionate relationships. . . . He will want to attain such a place more than anything else and may even forget that once, when he was hungry, he sneered at love."

Love Magic = Love Needs

The question I get most from people who ask for a reading is "when will love finally appear in my life?" This branch of magic is about all relationships and interactions with another being and the warmth they bring to your life. This is where romance, companionship, compassion, cooperation, understanding, acceptance, and a host of other emotionally supportive interactions live, as well as hurtful, bullying, gaslighting, and abusive interactions.

Maslow kind of skims over this level of need, yet I see it as one we get stuck on more than any other. His comments about this level focus on it being the reward for getting your shit together in the previous two levels and the "thwarting of the love needs as basic in the picture of maladjustment."

Thought leaders of 20th-century "success" schools push loving emotions away or deny that they are there because they make us too vulnerable. If you are vulnerable, you are no longer safe, and someone is out to get you. At the same time, we look at true or unconditional love as the savior and healer of it all. If it is not a fairy-tale ending, if it fails, it must not be true love. What a conundrum! *Love* becomes such an aspirational word that we can never reach its unconditional heights. We mere human beings will always come up short of the unconditional ideal, and that keeps us stuck in this energetic deficit.

Maslow may not have spent a lot of time on the love layer, but I spend a shit ton here as a magical consultant. This branch of the Magic 5 touches every person we interact with, making it kind of a big deal. Magic takes two people or beings to manifest, and that is what this level is all about. Any spell you cast will need one more person to manifest. You want a raise? You need your boss to approve it. Do you need inspiration? You need to hear, see, or experience something someone else has done to trigger that moment. You need a bunch of money? Someone has to spend it on you. You want a date? You need someone to show up. *Connection* is the catalyst to spark your magic into action.

In the English language, there are many words for affection but only one word for love, and that limits us in how we look at this branch of magic. Not every type of love spell is about Wesley and Buttercup's one true love, leaving us at a loss for words. The Greeks have six words for love that widen the playing field and make our relationship with relationships more well-rounded: *Eros* spells are about passion and sex. *Philia* spells are about deep friendship; *Ludus* spells are about playfulness. *Agape* spells are universal, unconditional love. *Pragma* spells are about long-standing love. *Philautia* spells are about self-love.

These love spell categories can be hived off again. Friendship spells can be used at work to help everyone function as a team. Family and home blessing spells call on that agape energy. Spells to build community fall in the love category since they fit right into Maslow's affectionate relationships.

Maslow's level of love bleeds deeply into the levels above and below it. Many relationship choices are made in relation to safety. Is the security the other person offers the draw? Do you stay in a toxic relationship because of financial insecurity? Do you stay in a toxic job because it pays well? Your magical needs bleed over to other branches as well. Rarely is a deficit in your energy myopically focused on one magical need, and generally there is a connection to another that is asking for a spellcasting boost.

The vast number of clinical studies around relationships have nothing on the number of love spells available with a quick internet search. The struggle with love and the need for love magic are the inspiration for music and a cornerstone of the blues. Love and relationships do indeed make rich men beg, good men sin, and tough men cry—we really know what it's like to sing the blues.

Love deficits bleed upward too: they call for healing and clearing so we can move from addiction and codependency into the self-love and acceptance needed to build self-esteem.

Healing and Clearing Magic = Esteem Needs

Getting to the esteem level of Maslow's hierarchy of needs means there has been some self-evaluation and you have found a bit of stability in the material world with your safety and in your relationships. Maslow describes our esteem needs as the impetus for "a stable, firmly based, (usually) high valuation of themselves, for self-respect, or self-esteem, and for the esteem of others." When we start feeling good about who we are and what we are up to, we feel good overall. He further describes this as "soundly based on real capacity, achievement and respect from others." In other words you are living a life based in reality and surrounding yourself with people who love and respect you and you them. *Wow*—life goals! These are amazing, but know that they live only in the moment you experience them. Your self-esteem is always on the roller-coaster ride: one day you feel amazing and the next you are struggling to find your worth. It's completely normal.

Maslow talks about self-esteem having two subsets, which I have named confidence and recognition. This is why I connect two branches of the Magic 5 to this level. *Healing* and *clearing* are similar yet different magical outcomes. Both are subtle, work specifically on the self, and are often overlooked. Still, they are two sides of the same coin, with healing being an internal process and clearing being an external one. Although they are connected to this higher level of Maslow's needs, their magic happens in tandem with all spells you are casting.

Self-esteem is created with each and every need that is met in love, safety, and physical issues; self-esteem is also destroyed when these levels are damaged by the circumstances around you. When you cast a candle spell, your confidence is *required* to power up your magic, and your confidence is *built* when that spell is successful. This level and these branches of magic are present in every magical intent you push out into the world and every empowered action you take to change your circumstances.

Healing of your internal process and beliefs is needed to resolve the love, protection, or prosperity issues that are inspiring your candle spell. When you are manifesting any spell, you may need to clear away the blocks and energetic sabotage in your way. Those blocks may be ones you placed in your path yourself or they may be from others; either way, they need to be cleared. This is why many traditions call on us to cleanse before we cast. Get rid of the junk that will hold you back and move into the mental and energetic space that supports your candle spell. Without these two branches of the Magic 5 you will be lighting candles for the same thing in different variations until your ceiling blacks with soot.

There is a bonus in working with healing and clearing magic in that you open the paths to creativity, to spirit, and to psychic abilities. You open the paths to communication, you find more tranquility, and you increase your sense of well-being. So all those other areas of magic we have talked about are covered with this level of work. When you light a candle for inspiration, you are clearing your doubt, healing your fear, and empowering your self-esteem. With this addition to every candle spell, your success rate increases.

Success of Your Spell = Self-Actualization

Self-actualization is the *bingo* of achieving your goals. I like to think of actualization as the last step to manifestation: you had an idea, added energy and action to it, faced your emotional issues around it, and made it a part of your everyday life. According to the Oxford Dictionary, *manifest* is defined as "to show something clearly, through signs or actions." *Actualize* is "to make something that could possibly happen or be achieved really happen or be achieved." Whether this is a magical process or a personal development process, you are experiencing similar results that often feel fleeting. As evolving humans and magical practitioners, we are always moving the goalpost to personal fulfillment, often without realizing and celebrating that leveling up.

During the preparation for Coventry's twentieth anniversary party, I was a wreck. I felt like a failure and an imposter. I thought, at twenty years in business I should own a Lexus and live in a McMansion. I was nowhere close to that. Personally, I had recently had my home foreclosed on due to the tanking market; my car was practical, basic, and aging; and I was still living paycheck to paycheck. Then there was the financial struggle we were still experiencing at Coventry. How could I feel successful with all this stacked against me?

During that time, I was cleaning my office for a paint job and found a New Year's declaration from 2007. I wrote that my measurement of success was to go grocery shopping without requiring coupons and to buy a book anytime I wanted to. Talk about success scope creep: I had moved from coupons to a Lexus and budgeting for a book to budgeting for a McMansion without recognizing what I had actualized and manifested along the way. I was shopping for small batches of groceries several times a week, and I had a library filled with books bought on a whim. Recognizing how far I had moved the goalpost in the previous five years allowed the twentieth anniversary to become an event of gratitude instead of judgment. Celebrating that I had leveled up my thought process, my business, and my comfort levels allowed me to start being and loving who I truly am. I stepped out of the energy of "should" and into the energy of "I am."

Maslow agrees that self-actualization is the process of discovering that satisfaction of doing what we are suited for. "A musician must make music, an artist must paint, a poet must write, if he is to be ultimately happy. What a man can be, he must be. This need we may call self-actualization." The satisfaction, empowerment, and feeling of connection to a greater power you feel when you watch a candle spell manifest in your life are unequaled. This power is what you hang on to in times of struggle; this power is what gives you courage and faith to try another spell and walk the uncomfortable path of evolution.

Maslow reminds us that we experience differing urgencies as life throws a variety of monkey-shit-filled issues at us. The Magic 5 combined with Maslow's hierarchy of needs gives you a few clues to dig deeper into the why of the candle spell you are crafting. For instance, if you have writer's block and need a blockbusting spell, what is the deeper need? Are you trying to connect to others? Are you facing a fear that makes you feel too vulnerable? Are you trying to sell your work? Maybe you need to clear the junk in your head and heal the doubt. When you dig in, you point your magic in the direction that will get you the fastest result.

I find that most modern psychology has roots deep in the spiritual world and its original magic. Maslow is no exception. He studied the spiritual philosophies of the Blackfoot tribe and Buddhism, and you can see their influence as well as how we come full circle back to the roots of magic.

TAKING A NEW
PERSPECTIVE ON MAGIC

You have traveled all this way through this exploration of the underpinnings of magic with me, and as a reward, I will give you a set of questions to ask yourself about your issue to get a new perspective on what magic you need. This is another way to get to the why of your spell. This process is best served with inquisitiveness. There is no right or wrong answer—there is only *your* answer.

What if, in all of your frustration and pain you are exactly where you need to be? If you feel strongly about something, you are buzzing with energy. It will fill and surround you with a generous amount of it. Tapping into the energy that already surrounds you and redirecting it into a magical solution is spiritual alchemy. An example of spiritual alchemy is when you tap into gratitude or dig for the lesson in the challenge and naturally shift your energy.

I call this my zen magic, and in all honesty it has taken me years to get to this place. I used to take things so personally and make all interactions about me. It is a normal and natural perspective to have because, of course, everything in your life is about you. It's when you realize that not everything in *other people's lives* is about you that this new perspective is available for use.

I came to understand this new perspective when I was writing all the cards for the Coventry Magic Oracle. I needed to show how any candle can be used for every magical branch of energy if you shift your perspective. For instance, if all you had was a Money Draw candle and you needed to work some clearing energy, how would that work? You can clear your energy by pushing out the negative vibes through pulling your feelings of confidence and abundance to the surface. This energy reminds your energy that there is no room for what limits you when you are feeling abundant. How does a banishing candle like Coventry's "Needed Change" bring love into your life? The new perspective is to banish the feelings of loneliness and the fear you have around love, making room for it to enter.

Real magic from your Aunt Jacki:
When I discovered that Coventry was being embezzled from, I was a wreck. I was angry and victimized and lost. This was exactly the reaction needed in that moment, and I let myself grieve all the betrayal and hurt until I was exhausted from it—for about two weeks. Once I released that initial hurt, I took a moment to ask myself what my new perspective would be. What was I going to do with all this energy of anger, loss, and betrayal? I dug deep to clear out old beliefs and behaviors. If I still felt somewhat profitable, even while someone was siphoning off cash from me every day, imagine the profit and feelings of success when that stopped. My new perspective was to take the energy of loss and send all of my limiting beliefs, bad behaviors, and old mental tapes with it into the spiritual burn pile to be transformed. I declared the statement "We have always done it that way" to be a sign to review the process and make it better. That new perspective allowed me to manifest double the amount that was stolen in sales, savings, and opportunities within ninety days. If I had stayed with the perspective of betrayal and victimhood, I would have still recovered, but much slower and filled with resentment that would continually keep my spirit small.

What could a new perspective on your biggest issue look like for you? It's nearly impossible to take on a new perspective when you are in the initial reactive response to the circumstances. Give yourself a moment to feel the justified feelings, knowing that you are not ready to take action yet. Taking action while you are reactive will lead to regret or a bigger problem. This is how witch wars get started, and everyone loses in a witch war. Acknowledging your feelings is the first and most important step in using your troubles to create solutions. Get them all out, and then use them as fuel for what's next.

Unpacking this new perspective takes a quick five questions, and the answers will help you supercharge your spell.

Grab your Candle Magic Journal and answer these questions as a warm-up to your "Why Is That?" exercise. Or maybe you'll want to answer these questions after the "Why Is That?" for getting a new perspective on confusing answers. You can do this to confirm what you discover about yourself or do this to ask powerful questions and change your world.

FIVE QUESTIONS TO UNCOVER YOUR DEEPER MAGICAL NEED

1. Does this issue affect my financial well-being, my stability, or a physical item? (Prosperity)

2. Does this need make me feel vulnerable or at risk in any way? (Protection)

3. Is this need influenced or affected by another person or group of people? (Love)

4. Am I looking to create a new path or avoid a block that was put in my path? Is there an obstacle that I keep running into? (Clearing)

5. Does this issue send me into anxiety just thinking about it? Do I trigger fear or inner resistance? (Healing)

The deficit in this deeper need is what has triggered your reactive response, so it is the new perspective that will use the rocket fuel of your emotions to create really powerful magic. Every yes you get when you ask those five questions tells you what magical energy you can bring into your spell to ensure its success.

In dealing with my embezzlement tale, I had three yeses. My situation was influenced by another person, affected my financial well-being, and was a trigger for many embedded fears. I brought all three of those energies into my spellwork, plus the energy of loss, and flipped the script. I used healing energy to find the triggers, fears, and beliefs in the love and prosperity branches of magic. Prosperity and love magic got powered up, and I was able to bring my whole Coventry team into the healing process. Every action and decision took us in the same direction to replace this money with new and to recover with profit. We did it, and I was able to share with each and every person the profit we generated. That in turn healed some staff-employer relationship fears I had.

BEING TERMINALLY UNIQUE

With everything in life, there are exceptions to the rule, but as a wise woman once told me, "If you live your life by the exceptions to the rule, the exceptions rule you." That is why every time I teach a new perspective class, I invite people to challenge me to fit their magical needs into the Magic 5. This is my favorite thing to do, and here are the best examples from those challenges:

Home blessing: What is causing the need for a home blessing? That perspective defines which of the Magic 5 you will turn to. Are you moving into a new house? You are using clearing and healing magic. Are there lots of arguments in the house? You are using love magic. Are you needing to renovate do you want to stop a money pit flow of needed repairs? That is prosperity magic.

Psychic development: When you open your psychic centers and work in mastering the skills of these spiritual muscles, it is a blend of clearing and healing magic. You are clearing out the judgment and limitations of the logical world and healing the beliefs and blocks they created.

Your son is in legal trouble? Protection and clearing. Then healing after he wins the court case.

You want to command someone to do as you say? Love—it is a relationship that you are controlling.

Communication spell? Are you clearing the channels of communication? That is clearing magic. Are you healing past arguments? Healing magic. Connecting with your customers? Prosperity magic. Connecting with your staff or coworkers? Love magic with clearing magic.

Psychic connections, talking to the dead, or spiritual inspiration? Love magic if you are building a relationship with a spirit. Clearing to open up your psychic centers. Protection if you are ensuring you don't get jumped by a spirit you are communicating with. All three will be triple effective!

Challenge yourself with your own magical needs and ask the Magic 5 questions. You will then understand where your starting point is.

SETTING INTENT

Why doesn't the universe already know what you want? You have been complaining about the thing enough—you would think your guides would just give you what you want. For that matter, shouldn't God or one of your guides know what is best for you and just make it happen? The answer is no. You have free will, and that means your brain is cluttered with all the ideas you have ever had—good and bad. You are scanning through a million possibilities before you even get out of bed. How in the world would the divine know what you really mean and want in all that mess?

Since your mind is going a gazillion miles a second, it's hard to pin down what you really want on the fly. It's like choosing one ice cream at a place that has 100 flavors: there are so many options, including whether or not you should have any in the first place. Sometimes you know exactly what you want, and boom—intent set and ice cream scooped. Sometimes they are out of your fave flavor and you are in the mood for something different. You have to start eliminating what you *don't* want and making a list of what you *do* want. Then you have to assess everything you do want and decide what option you want *the most*. Do you try something new or keep safe with a variation of your favorite? What about those sherbets in the corner, or the dairy- and sugar-free option? Cone or bowl, waffle or cake cone? If you go into the ice cream shop and yell, "Give me ice cream that is good!" who are you going to be mad at when you get a mess that you don't even recognize? You are going to be mad at yourself—you are the responsible party here because you didn't tell the universal ice cream scooper what you really wanted. Defining what you want and declaring your intention is 100 percent your responsibility. No one is going to do it for you. No internet meme, TED Talk, song, therapist, or well-meaning advice from a friend can set your intention. They don't have your history, perspective, or issues. Only you have that powerful tool.

Setting intentions is like goal setting for your spirit. An intention is more empathic than logical, and your spirit responds to the emotion that drives your intention more than the logic that drives a goal. The universe likes logic; your spirit likes the emotion. Together, you can create big magic.

Modern business and success books have picked up on the power of intention setting and talk about its importance before you ever define a goal. Intentions align your goals with your spiritual and emotional motivations. That is: if you don't give yourself a good enough reason to walk through the tough parts, you won't finish.

The intention you set needs to be a bigger emotional commitment than the issue that you are overcoming with your magic. As your spell progresses, having your intention clear in your head fuels it toward completion and opens your spirit to receive what you are manifesting. It also reminds you to look for proof along the way.

CLARIFYING YOUR INTENT—GETTING OUT OF THE SHOULDS

The "Why Is That?" exercise is the best way to clarify your intent and get to the core of what you really want. It gets you past the "shoulds" and into your true desire. Once you do all the steps of setting an intent, building your words of power, choosing your candle, finding the right time, adding your accessories, and setting up your space, will you get what you ask for? Maybe.

Did you ask for the right thing? Is it what you really want? It's difficult to be certain of asking for what we really want when we are conditioned to *not* ask for what we want. It's polite to turn down the second slice of pie or tell your company you don't need help setting the table. We are inundated with social media that tells us what we *should* want and aspire to. Even self-help books zero in on how to be successful according to their own definition of success.

I have been driven for years by the shoulds in the world. I should be thin. I should have a million-dollar business. I should be the perfect mother, the perfect daughter. I should be organic, vegan, sustainable, pretty, pristine, casual, put together, relaxed, driven, fantastic, crafty, passionate, compassionate, tolerant, accountable, have boundaries . . . and more.

Ursula Adams, founder of SheHive *(theshehive.com)*, writes a blog at the first of every year about the lies of the shoulds. "I Google 'things I should do every day' every December (and took the results off the first page) . . . In 2018 the list returned 72 results. In 2019, it jumped to 234 and in 2020 there were a whopping 338 things we should be doing every day (thanks to a man named Frank)! This year, luckily, the experts are only suggesting we do 269 daily." Adams has found that aspiring to things you should do every day causes depression and a feeling of failure. When she broke free of them and focused on how she wanted to *be*, her life took a turn toward joy.

Staying stuck in this mindset of should can crash a spell.

Your should doesn't align your energy with what your soul really needs.

You will always manifest what you believe before you manifest what you want.

What you want isn't always what you need for your candle spell to be successful.

What you really need tends to go to the bottom of the list of what your spirit is aligned with because you are stuck in the shoulds.

Shoulds create a vicious circle of sabotage.

Grab your Candle Magic Journal and revisit your "Why Is That?" notes. Look for the real intent that aligns with your spirit and soul, and start there. If that intent isn't quickly apparent, ask yourself the questions below and dive into your why from a new direction.

Take a moment right now and think about the next spell you want to cast.

A real-life example from your Aunt Jacki: I went through a three-year entrepreneurial training where the intent was to teach you how to get to $1 million in revenue. The program was great, no complaints. The intent seemed exactly what I should aspire to. I added in my candle magic on my prosperity altar with big goals. I told everyone about it and expected that we would all get aligned with manifesting this. My spell helped me find opportunities and hire people I thought would get me there. Yet in the end it all drove me to misery. The deals eventually fell through; the staff members would leave or become an unhealthy addition to my company. My sales did grow, but not to $1 mil, and the stress was not sustainable. I finally sat down with my partner and started to question why we wanted to get to $1 mil in revenue. The answer was to be successful. Why would we feel successful with $1 mil? Because that would bring stability to our business and we could pay our staff (and ourselves) more. Why is that important? Because we would have less stress about our personal finances. In the end creating joy.

Why do you want that?

Whose voice do you hear in your head when you think about that spell?

Is it your mother's voice, your teacher's voice, or someone else?

Does it come from your higher/divine self or from your ego?

Do you understand why you want that?

What does fulfillment look like?

Now, let's look at what motivates this clarified want:

How do you want to feel when this want is fulfilled?

What does that feeling mean to you?

What does that feeling validate or heal?

Why do you need that healing or validation?

Right there: that last answer is the basis of your intent. Then you build your intent statement from the bottom up and compare it to your initial idea. Is this still what you want?

There are several ways to write your intent and words of power, from stories to rhymes to daily affirmations. It's worth it to write them all in alignment to transform your spell into a new belief.

> We flipped the intent of our candle magic from manifesting revenue to "being a joyful, financially stable business that supports our staff with a living wage." That intent changed everything. My charms and words of power were different. My emotional commitment was stronger. And we moved forward in a healthy and sustainable way that kept us focused in having quality of life for everyone. The stress of status went away, and real opportunities aligned with our goal came into being. We crossed the $1 mil threshold within twenty-four months and have the joyful energy to keep going and growing.

TURNING YOUR INTENT INTO SOMETHING TO BELIEVE IN

Words of power tell a story of success and create a belief. When you step into an emotionally charged assumption or conclusion and revisit that story again and again, you are creating a belief. We manifest what we believe before any intention we may set. It's hard to override an embedded belief, so take the time to make that belief one that works to your benefit.

There is a rhythm to writing out your intent so it becomes a belief. It begins with writing in the past tense as if it has already happened. This perspective allows you to connect with the emotions that trigger a belief creation. It also will keep you motivated and give you clues on what your words of power for the spell will be. When you paint the picture of the outcome and beyond, you will find yourself celebrating sooner rather than later. Your words of power help you hold that vision, reaffirm your belief, and keep out of the doubt and fear that will crash your spell.

Give your spell the boundaries of a time frame. Goals without a time frame are just wishes. Seriously, how many papers got written because you were on a deadline? How many times were you able to clean your house top to bottom in an hour because guests were on their way? Give your magic a due date that is attainable in the real world, and the spirits will help you meet that deadline and maybe even speed it up if they can.

Another real-life example from your Aunt Jacki: In the late spring of 2020, one of my ride-or-die friends was in a debilitating crisis. Their partner became deathly ill during the high point of the COVID-19 pandemic. Was it COVID? Was it organ failure? What was it!? They were inconsolable and could not get out of the fear. Together we constructed a spell with the intent of their partner coming home and returning to health. I asked what the ideal outcome for the situation would be. I asked for the story of what it would look like to bring their partner home. I had them describe the scene as I wrote it down. What would happen when they went to the hospital to pick their partner up? What would the ride home be like? What would happen when they came into the house? What would occur in the following five days, thirty days, and three months? All of these details went onto the paper, and we used that as the focal point for the spell. We created a belief that this was how it would work out in the end. We created words of power as a daily intention to bring focus and an affirmation to be said multiple times in the day to bring peace. There were candles, oils, sprays, stones, symbols, etc. None of this was a replacement for good medical care. What we created first was a new belief that brought clarity and balanced emotions. This new calm allowed my bestie to be mentally present for their partner. They became a medical advocate for their partner and were able to prevent a big mistake that would have been irreversible. Creating the new belief built upon intent, story, focus, and words of power in the form of an affirmation was what made the rest of the magic work. Their partner came home the way the story described. It wasn't exact, but close enough to notice and be impressed by the story that was written.

Define what the signs of success are. *I will know that this spell is working when I (see, hear, feel) _____.* Using the example of my bestie, we defined success as "I will know this spell is successful when I hear our song on the radio." I have also used feelings to define success. "I will know this spell is working when I can let go of the outcome and feel free of the fear."

As your spell begins to show you the signs that it is on the right track, step into gratitude and give thanks to the spirits that assisted you. Seriously, this is really important. Do not take any of these energies for granted or they won't show the willingness to work hard for you in the future. Everything you put into your spell—especially gratitude—is energy that the spirits can use to manifest your spell, including the thanks you give to them.

Putting it all together looks like this:

I am so grateful to have _____ in my life. It was completed by _____ and I knew once _____ happened, I was on the right track. I am so thankful to _____ for helping me with this success of this spell.

I put a spell together for my daughter when she traveled to Japan. This was not a trip where I could hop on a plane and rescue her if something happened, and I was more nervous than I let on. I crafted a safe-travel spell and anointed her luggage and passport. I built words of power that clarified my intent in a successful way. Here's an example of how I created a spell using this past-tense method.

I am so grateful my daughter had an amazing experience in Japan. Her travels were interesting, exciting, and safe. She learned so much and is enriched by the experience. When she came home, she was tired and happy, and I was so happy to see her. I knew she was OK and having a good time when people asked me how she was doing and when she sent me messages over Facebook. I'm so grateful that our ancestors watched over her and thank them for their care of her body and spirit.

My daughter came home safe and sound and had had a life-changing experience. Was it because of the spell? I can't lay claim to that, but the spell certainly helped me to stay calm and focused on the happy ending of the story.

This process is not new, nor is it exclusive to the magical community. Imagine my inner glee when almost every entrepreneurial class I've been in had us start with the exercise of telling our future story as if it had already happened. I have written out my goals and intent, videoed my story, told it to 100 people, and was held accountable to it all while telling the story as if it had already happened. And I did manifest everything I declared. For this book, I revisited a future success story I wrote when I was in the Goldman Sachs 10,000 Small Businesses program. In 2017 I created a growth plan to enter a new market and grow revenue. I talked about an expanded staff, larger facilities, and a calmer life. Well, we did it. The 2021 revenue matched the numbers I defined in my growth plan. It didn't happen the way I envisioned, but the conclusion manifested with the intent and success story I wrote out. The vision I created was attainable and yet outside of my comfort zone. It involved identifying the right opportunities and doing the hard work that made them successful. That plan was not sitting on my altar with candles as a spell, but instead told to a group of 300 people so they all got excited with me. That collective energy added to the emotional commitment I made to the vision I wrote out and created a belief that this was possible. Public storytelling is a ceremony of sorts and in this case transformed it into a belief that my divine allies recognized and helped me manifest.

Magic is everywhere you look for it! Write your story of success. From this foundation, you can fine-tune your ingredients, craft your words of power, and grow your spell into transformational magic.

SPELLS, RHYMES, AFFIRMATIONS, AND WORDS OF POWER

Your candle spell needs your words to activate it. These words must be spoken aloud and tap into your belief in your power to cocreate magic with divinity. When you align your words of power with the keywords in your "Why Is That?" and add the fun of rhyme, you are crafting an incantation to break through any blocks and fears to manifesting new possibilities.

Spells That Rhyme

Why do all the best spells rhyme? Because they call to your inner child that believes in magic and the possibilities it holds. Rhymes also take us out of the serious logical world and into a place where not everything is as it seems, where a bit of preposterous chaos is at work. Think about when you were learning playground rhymes for the first time. What did they mean? What was going to happen to Mary Mack after she saw the elephants? Who is going to stink after the cork falls out of the bottle of ink? When we were kids, the rhymes helped us find order in a chaotic place where we needed to learn to take turns and work together. The rhythm of the rhyme triggers our memory muscles and promotes language development through repetition.

In magic, rhyme activates your inner child, who is a catalyst to your magic. You are inviting them into your magic, welcoming them to be delighted and ridiculous with you. Rhyming spells call up a bit of chaos and re-form it into the energy that will help manifest your goal and believe all of it is possible. Also, rhymes just *feel* magical and true. If you were picked to be *it* by a rhyming song, there was no arguing the fate.

> *Inka-dink, a bottle of ink, the cork fell out, and you stink. Not because you're dirty, not because you're clean, just because you kissed the girl behind the magazine. And . . . you . . . are . . . it.*

Get transported to the clapping game of Mary Mack and how magical it was to go all the way to the end without missing a handclap. That was a total win!

> *Miss Mary Mack, Mack, Mack*
> *All dressed in black, black, black*
> *With silver buttons, buttons, buttons*
> *All down her back, back, back.*
>
> *She asked her mother, mother, mother*
> *For 50 cents, cents, cents*
> *To see the elephants, elephants, elephants*
> *She jumped the fence, fence, fence.*
>
> *She jumped so high, high, high*
> *She reached the sky, sky, sky*
> *And didn't come back, back, back*
> *'Til the 4th of July, ly, ly!*
>
> *Miss Mary Mack, Mack, Mack*
> *All dressed in black, black, black*
> *With silver buttons, buttons, buttons*
> *All down her back, back, back.*
>
> *She asked her mother, mother, mother*
> *For 50 cents, cents, cents*

To see the elephants, elephants, elephants
She jumped the fence, fence, fence.

She jumped too low, low, low
She stubbed her toe, toe, toe
and that's the end of our show, show, show.

We even used rhymes as our first charm spells:

I'm rubber, you're glue. Everything you say bounces off me and sticks to you.

When I write the spells for the Coventry candles, I have to get a little silly and call up my inner child. I need her since I can't write a spell if I am serious or stressed. I set the mood of play and fun that entices her. Starting with my warm-up, I will write the most ludicrous thing I can think of, maybe a dirty limerick or two. As I let go of the logical world, I can dive into my couplets and create rhymes in sets of two that become the eight-line spells that grace my products. There is a standard rhythm to my spells:

Two lines for what I am manifesting

Two lines for calling on assistance

Two lines for clearing out limits

Two lines for reaffirming what I am manifesting and closing the spell

This format is the opening guideline, and then I get creative and use poetic license. Looking at the following money spells I have written, you'll see I mix up the order and add or subtract a few lines, but they still hit all the points and have proven to be successful.

From Coventry's Blessed Herbal Money Draw Candle
I open the path to wealth without end.
The money I need the universe will send.
Bills will be paid, my coffers overflow,
My worries released, my wealth will grow.
My own blocks be they from spirit or mind,
no longer hamper, no longer bind.
Harming none and helping all is how it shall be.
This I make true. 3x3x3

From Coventry's Blessed Prosperity Candle
This Candle so sweet I hold before me,
ignites the seeds of prosperity.
I call on forces higher than I,
to awaken the wealth that I hold inside.
May I be enriched in the most correct way,
harming none and helping all as it fills my stay.
I call on thee in perfect trust and love,
to create abundance from above.
This I make true and so it will be,
bring what is needed times three.

From Coventry's Prosperity Quick Spell (retired)
Cash, cash, in you flow.
Into my pockets money grows
Paper, coin, or checks to cash
Getting ever larger, my money stash
Protect the fund and keep me wise
My bad money habits are neutralized
This I make true, so it will be
Money magic is cast 3x3x3

Try your own rhyming words of power. Get into the mood by getting ridiculous. Listen to children's songs, sing old rhymes from your childhood, watch humorous cartoons, and write with crayons and markers in bold colors. The more you play in this way, the easier and more creative it will get.

Affirmations

Rhyming spells are amazing for lifting your spirit and mind into the world of possibilities.

Affirmations are amazing for the logical mind, reprogramming your thought process on a quantum level. Affirmations are a simple, repeatable, and powerful magical tool. They are more approachable and believable, especially for those who hate rhyming (*GASP!*). If the affirmation powers you up more than a rhyme, you are an affirmation person.

Affirmations are written in present or past tense, just like writing the story of your intent. Writing your affirmation in future tense might get you stuck in an energetic loop. In essence you are affirming that you will always be looking for the thing to manifest.

"I *will manifest* prosperity in every action" is future tense and tells your spirit that you have not done the thing yet, but you plan on it . . . someday. When you do the thing, it's going to be great, but you are not doing the thing right now. "I *manifest* prosperity in every action" is present tense and tells your spirit that you are doing the thing right now and the manifestation of it is immanent and the check is in the mail.

"Every action I have taken has brought me prosperity" is a past tense that tells your spirit that you already did the thing and are harvesting your rewards right now—no need to pass go because your $200 is here, in Monopoly game terms.

Affirmations are only in the positive. The universe is not ironic and does not understand the negative. Be literal and specific: "I won't be poor" is not positive. I won't = I am. When you craft your affirmation, check its level of positivity by putting *I am* in front of the sentence.

"I am free of poverty" is borderline negative. You are still talking about poverty. If there is a negative mindset to heal, it will be normal to write your affirmation in that way.

"I am wealthy in body, mind, and spirit, and it is growing in every way" is positive in every way. Notice the word *and*. Never use *but*, which negates everything in the beginning of the sentence and only allows for the thoughts that come after.

Affirmations are active. If at all possible, give your phrase movement and action. For instance "I am wealthy in body, mind, and spirit" is finished, complete. "I am wealthy in body, mind, and spirit, and it is growing in every way" gives it room for more growth.

Affirmations are specific. The affirmation we have been looking at, "I am wealthy in body, mind, and spirit, and it is growing in every way," is not specific enough. If you are growing in every way, you may need to get a bigger belt. "I am wealthy in body, mind, and spirit, and my financial fortune is growing every day" makes it specific.

Affirmations are simple and fast to make. Start with an *I am* statement, add a dynamic emotional statement in the positive, and make sure it is active.

I release the limiting thoughts that block my prosperity. I open my mind, heart, and being to the unlimited abundance of the universe.

This Coventry prosperity affirmation is active with the intention to release, be open, and be unlimited. It is very effective, and I get comments about how people still use the affirmation all on its own after the candle is consumed.

Affirmations can accompany a rhyming spell to keep the spell top of mind and empowered until it manifests. Repeating the rhyming spell every day and then affirming it throughout the day expand what you are asking and bring your spirit into alignment with the desired outcome.

For example, set up a simple happy home candle spell like this.

Light a Blessed Herbal Happy Home candle, and say the rhyming spell:

I call on forces higher than I to awaken the gifts that I hold inside.
To have a Happy Home that flows with love, is what I ask to create from
above.
May this come to me in the most correct way, bringing peace and serenity to
my day.
I call on thee in perfect love and trust, working with me, sending what is
just.
Harming none and helping all is how it shall be. This I make true. 3x3x3

Repeat an affirmation throughout the day that assumes success of your spell:

My home is abundant with blessings and love of the universe.
All who reside here are filled with peace and recognize and release tension as
it arises.

Can you see how that affirmation validates the spell and keeps your mind, emotions, and spirit in alignment with its success? It is also easier to remember and repeat multiple times a day. However you decide to write your spell, though, it's yours. It will be imperfect at best so embrace that! It will work for *you* because it is filled with *your* emotion and intent. It takes the chaos of the million ideas and distills it down to a focal point. Doing the spell is 100 percent more powerful than analyzing it to death. Make it good, and next time make it better.

When to Use Your Words of Power

Your intention, purpose for your ingredients, incantation, spell, and/or affirmation are all your words of power. They are activated only when you state them out loud. In your head they can only circle around, unproductive, until your inner saboteur convinces you this is crap. Spells are not actualized through thought, they are actualized through action with the first one being stating your spell out loud, and being proud while voicing it, dammit. Say it with conviction, confidence, and belief. If you don't believe it, why would the energies of the universe align to cocreate with you? Even if you have to be discreet about your spell, you can still speak quietly with the attitude and conviction you need.

Leverage the time and effort you put into turning your deeper need into words of power by repeating them throughout the spell. For the simplest spell, you can light the candle and say the words. Done and done—carry on with your day. If you have created an involved spell where you are doing a magical craft project, setting up an altar, and relighting your candle for several days, repeat those words of power throughout your spell to stay focused and energized.

The beginning, middle, and end of your spell can be punctuated by stating your intention, purpose, and incantation. This becomes a natural build to your energy, intensifying your magical power. State your intent as you are setting up your altar to give it purpose. Talk to the herbs and oils as you make your candle-dressing blend, giving your ingredients instructions and aligning them with your intent. Tell your story and state your words of power as you place your candles, repeating this again as you light them. Every time you repeat your spell, it builds the power to a peak level that aligns your body, mind, and spirit with the creative forces of the universe.

The number of times you say your incantation can become a part of the magic. Odd numbers leave room for your spell to grow. Saying your words of power three times as a quick build brings everything into alignment. Saying your words of power five times pushes past some of your blocks and fears. Saying your words of power seven times is very lucky. Saying your words of power nine times aligns you with the cocreative forces of the divine, overrides your doubts and fears, opens you up to expansion of your spell, and frees you of limitations.

Saying your words of power an even number of times aligns the energy with a group of people. This is more foundational and helps your spell take root. Saying your words of power four times creates a union between opposing forces and establishes a foundation. Saying your words of power six times brings love, cooperation, and peace. Saying your words of power eight times brings stability and helps them grow roots.

Repeat your words of power throughout your day to help the manifestation speed up. When you are physically away from your candle spell—and have extinguished the flame—writing your affirmation multiple times in the day, then saying it out loud will keep your spell charged with magic. The number of times you repeat your words of power and the time of day you say them can add to your magic. Sunrise, noon, sunset, midnight, 3 p.m., and 3 a.m. are powerful times to repeat your words of power, as are the number of the hour and whether the hands on the clock are going up or down.

Every time you relight your candle, restate your incantation at least once out loud to reaffirm your spell. Repeating the incantation the same number of times you originally committed to creates a groove in your spiritual record, confirming that every level of you is committed to the outcome of this spell.

Petition Papers

Your petition paper is what you write your words of power on. This object becomes part of your spell, and you can use it to expand the spell. When you are starting the spell, saying and repeating your words of power, it is important that you place that paper under or around your candle to connect its energy to the spell. This is different from any pictures or personal concerns you add to your candle magic ritual. You may end up writing on the picture or document to direct your magic, yet having a separate petition paper with your words of power is critical, even if you are repeating the same thing on the picture.

Your petition paper, once connected to your spell, can travel with you. You can repeat your words of power as you are holding the petition paper, sending the energy through the paper back to your spell. You can burn or destroy the petition paper as part of your spell. You can hold on to the petition paper after the candle is consumed to keep the energy going. You can also add that petition paper to a new spell. Whatever you decide to do, record it in your Candle Magic Journal.

CASTING FOR GUIDANCE

Trusting your intuition is great, and getting it confirmed by a divination tool is very empowering as it starts to create a greater trust in the direction of your candle magic. Divining for the higher purpose of your magic confirms your inner intuition and gives you a new perspective on the energy of your spell. It is also a safety valve if you are heading in the wrong direction.

Before I cast a big spell, I go in front of my spirit allies and ancestors and ask for their permission and support for my magical work. I have developed my own system with my spirit team over the years that gives me a yes or no. I also have a way for them to tell me to look deeper, to get help. You will develop your own intuitive tells with candle magic, especially if you start with basic tools and guidebooks to check in. Consider this your latest guidebook.

TAROT—WHY WING IT WHEN YOU CAN ACCESS THE WISDOM OF THE AGES?

Tarot not only tells the tale of your past; it is also a magical portal to create the vibration for your future. Centuries of intention, meaning, and empowerment surround the tarot so that by looking at a card you can bring its vibration to you. Try this experiment: Pull the Sun card from any deck and hold in between your palms. Feel as tension drains from your body and you become lighter and filled with energy. This is the magic of tarot. Each card has a vibrational signature that tunes in to your energetic state and gives you insight into the blind spot of what you don't want to or cannot see. When you are prepping a candle spell, you are looking to resolve what is in your blind spot. Really, if you knew what was in your blind spot, you would already understand what action to take. Use tarot to bring your deeper issue to light and either let go of the spell or craft it into big magic. Refer to the index in the back of the book to look at more specific vibrations of each card in prosperity, protection, love, clearing, and healing spells.

Using Tarot for Your "Why Is That?" Exercise

Blind spots are powerful tools our ego uses to protect us from what is scary or goes against our beliefs. We can interpret and justify any actions and reactions in our life as necessary. Remember how you don't want to be the bad guy in your own story? That is what your blind spot can shield you from. It can also shield you from information you aren't ready to handle. When you have several reasons for this blind spot, it becomes a habit.

Use the "Why Is That?" exercise to look into that darkness to understand your deeper need. What if that place is too damn scary to look into—the monsters are too real and your subconscious overrules your primal brain and says, "*Nope*, nothing to see here, move along"? If that place is that damn scary, grab your tarot cards and do the variation of the "Why Is That?" spread from *Coventry Magic*. This dive into your why deals with your hidden or blind spot thoughts, emotions, and intuition.

For tarot definitions, use your favorite tarot guide or the booklet that comes with the deck.

"Why Is That?" Tarot Spread

Prep your paper the same way described in the "Why Is That?" exercise on page 12 and write out the challenge you need magical assistance

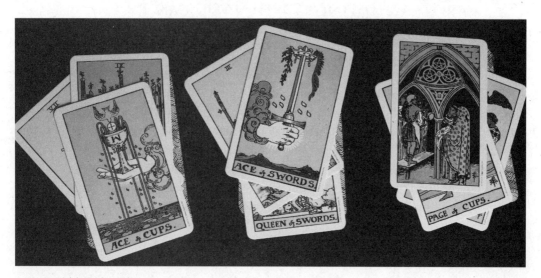

1. Your Hidden Thoughts
2. Your Hidden Feelings
3. Your Hidden Intuition

with. Set up your reading space with intention and respect. Grab your deck and start shuffling while thinking about the issue you are crafting your candle spell for. Every card you draw is about you and your energy. It's how you see things on the primal and unconscious levels and what is in your blind spot. At no point is any card, court or otherwise, talking about the specific behavior of another person. It is talking about how *you* feel or perceive the other person. It's all about you, babe.

Current Situation: Either choose the card that best describes your current situation or cut the shuffled deck in the middle and draw a card for this. The card you randomly draw from the deck is your deep feelings about the challenge at hand. When you read the meaning of this card, look for words that you resonate with. Write those words under your challenge.

Reshuffle the deck and cut it into three piles. Flip over the card on the top of the pile farthest to your left. Flip the top card over in each consecutive pile to the right. Don't turn the next card over until you've written down your thoughts about the previous one:

- Why #1—Your hidden thoughts: This is what is on the surface of your struggle. These are the thoughts that pass like ninjas through your mind, changing your mood and influencing your choices. Go to the first why section on your paper and write the keywords, meaning, and your initial thoughts about this card.

- Why #2—Your hidden feelings: These are the feelings about the situation that you have buried because they are too much, you are not ready for them, or they challenge your current belief about the situation. Move to the second why section and write down the keywords, definition, and your initial reaction to this card.

- Why #3—Your hidden intuition: This is what you know intuitively about the situation but are not willing to look at. This is the thing that is bothering you and you don't know why. Move to the third why and write down the keywords, definition, and initial response to this card.

These cards may seem to pull you away from the original problem. They may not make sense to you, but there *is* a message there for you. Review your notes and look for a repeating pattern, words, or reactions. Underline the words that stand out to you and that resonate. Read just those words and see what comes to you.

Take this reading deeper by pulling the next card in the pile, one position at a time. Record the keywords and the definition that stick out to you in the appropriate why position in your notes. This second layer is deep enough to show you why you feel that way, what is motivating you, and how you need to address it. These keywords are also clues to the candles, ingredients, and words of power that will enhance the spell you are crafting.

If you are still feeling stuck, identify *one word* for each card and write your why story from there. Play with your intuition and hold a card between your palms to feel your reaction, noting any words or images that come to mind.

Repercussions Tarot Spread

This spread gives you a bit of insight into the potential results of the candle spell you are planning at this moment. Every spell you cast affects you first, your environment next, and your target last. This is a great check-in to see if your intention is clear and if the spell will go the same way in life as you've pictured it in your mind.

Give a good shuffle to the cards while thinking about your goal, your ingredients, and the target of this spell. Cut the deck and pull the trajectory card and interpret it. Reshuffle the deck and cut it into three piles: how it affects you, how it affects your environment, and how it affects the target. Flip the top card of each pile one at a time and interpret. For tarot definitions, use your favorite tarot guide or the booklet that comes with the deck.

> **The trajectory of your spell:** this is your hidden intention. If this card shows that your hidden intention is far from what you think your intention is, don't do the spell. Go back to the earlier exercises and keep digging to uncover your deeper need and work on healing yourself first. *If you are curious about the spell you are not going to do, finish the reading to see the outcome with the promise that you will not do the spell.*

> **How it affects you:** What will change or react within you. When you cast a spell, it comes from you and your energy evolves to make the spell

possible. If you are doing a prosperity spell, you evolve to vibrate in a way that will bring prosperity. If you are doing a revenge spell, you will evolve to vibrate in a way that will exact that result. Not all spells are good or bad, but they all are an evolution of energy.

How it affects your environment: You live in your environment. When you evolve and change vibrations, your environment will react to that. It will either shift to harmonize with your change or become discordant and create chaos. You could cast that protection spell, and your friend group leaves because they don't have your best interest at heart—true story!

How it affects your target: This card is the one that tells you if your spell will be effective. If the card you pull is far from your intended result, pull two more cards from that pile: the first to ask what changes are needed, and the second to see the results to the change suggested. If this is not a good result, do not do the spell. Go back to your why, or do the "Why Is That?" exercise to find what you really need to do.

Don't judge the results of this reading, just go with the flow and you may avoid disastrous potential consequences. I have avoided negative consequences with this reading, and I have also created disastrous consequences when I didn't do this reading and went off on an emotional tear. The spell worked amazingly, and it tore apart my life as a repercussion. I got through it, but a few things were forever changed.

Tarot is the most detailed divination you can do to forecast the success of your spell. There are also faster methods that are worth testing and playing with as you build your own system.

ORACLE DECKS—BREAKING FROM THE STATUS QUO

I am a sucker for a good oracle deck. (I even created my own Coventry Magic Oracle.) I love how each deck takes you on a different journey with a different set of spirits guiding you. Imagine how a favored oracle deck can lead you to a deeper understanding of the repercussions of your spell. Oh, the insight! Tarot purists will look down on an oracle as a poor copy. I look at an oracle as the divine speaking through the artist and author for a specific purpose, as tarot can be a little rigid in its interpretation. I don't know about you, but

I have been reading tarot for so long I can easily jump to conclusions about what a card means. I will use an oracle in times when I am highly emotional about a subject and desperate for a specific outcome. I am a master at tricking myself, and most people I meet seem to be good at that as well.

When you are getting ready to read with your oracle, treat it the same way you would your tarot deck. Use the same spreads outlined in the tarot section before this. You will have to intuit your own reference as to what candle or spell each card is pointing you toward. An oracle desk is excellent for use in the "Why Is That?" reading as most oracles speak directly to your higher self. You will most likely be looking up the meanings of each card in the instruction book and can pull out your keywords from there.

No matter what type of deck you use to divine the outcome of your spell, play a little! Have fun, and if you get confused, check your results with the pendulum or a coin toss for a definitive yes or no.

PENDULUMS—THE TATTLETALES OF YOUR HIGHER SELF

What is a pendulum? For divination, in a very broad sense, it is a weighted object at the base of a string or chain. Subtle changes in your body, the energy that surrounds you, and the influence of spirits can affect the movement of the pendulum when it is held from a fixed position. Even a pendulum suspended in a cage can show movement from the telekinetic energy around it.

I see pendulums as akin to muscle testing where your higher or divine self is using the subtle twitches of your muscles to influence the movement of the pendulum. It can be hard to hear the voice of our higher and our primal self through all the noise of everyday life, so using a pendulum is a fast track to your inner voice.

You are always sensing more energy around you than your rational mind is taking in, and a pendulum can communicate what is beyond your rational viewpoint in your extrasensory perception. Spirits, disruptive energy, energy that aligns with you, and even the effect of the food you are about to eat can be perceived through your extra senses and communicated through your pendulum. Divining for your candle spell before, during, and after with a pendulum taps into your ESP; you can check if the spell you are proposing is aligned with your highest good, if the candle spell is going as expected, and if it influenced the results you are looking for. Intuitively, you know all of these answers; your higher self is just itching to give them to you through your pendulum.

When using your pendulum to test for your candle spell, follow these best practices:

Picking your pendulum: If you have one, the more you use it, the more accurate it will be. When you are new to using a pendulum, picking one is strictly by preference. Become acquainted with the energy of your new divination tool by asking yes and no questions you already have the answers to. Not having a pendulum is not a problem either. Use a necklace or a ring hanging on a chain that you regularly wear as they will be already in tune with your energy.

Holding the pendulum: Hold the chain between your thumb and forefinger, draping the chain over your finger with about 6 inches of room below. Brace your wrist against a steady object and get comfortable: you are going to be here for a while. As you tire, the answers of your pendulum reading will lose their accuracy.

Preparing the questions: Be specific, clear, and concise and bring up only one question at a time. Ask only yes or no questions. The best questions are under ten words long. With more than ten, you will forget what you said and it's probably two questions. The examples below are a bit general; be specific to your situation.

- "Is this spell for my highest good?"
- "Will a love spell bring _____ back to me?"
- "Will this money spell solve my cash flow issue?"
- "Will this protection spell stop what is making me feel unsafe?"
- "Will this revenge spell go back to the person who is doing me harm?"

If you are doing something complicated, write it down on paper in steps with a desired outcome and ask if the spell you are planning will bring the results described on the paper.

Keep your question list small. Your arms and shoulders will fatigue, and your answers will get skewed.

Opening up to the reading: Take several calming breaths and use your favorite grounding technique to get centered. Invite your higher self to talk to you through your pendulum by asking easily established yes and no questions. Ask your higher self to rotate the pendulum clockwise when it is fully aligned with you and your pendulum.

Interpreting the movements

- YES: Up and down, perpendicular to your body. Always confirm your yes answers by asking another way.

- NO: Side to side, parallel to your body. No means no.

You may also get the indications listed below:

- HUH? Or UNCLEAR: Standstill or angle responses are neither yes or no. Your question is unclear, incomplete, or inconclusive.

- Energy coming to you: Clockwise circles. The wider the circle, the more or the faster it will be coming in.

- Energy moving away: Counterclockwise circles. The wider the circle, the more or the faster it will be leaving.

If these indicators don't speak to you, make up your own. Be consistent with the same movement interpretation every time or you will confuse yourself on every level.

Asking the questions: Start with a prayer of gratitude for your spirit allies, ancestors, and guardians for guiding and protecting you. Invite your higher self and gatekeeper spirit to send the answers for your questions through the pendulum. Still your pendulum between each question.

- Ask if your higher self is ready and willing to answer your questions with truth and in your highest good.

- Ask if your gatekeeper/guardian is able to keep out any negative or dishonest influences.

- If you get a yes on all these questions, ask if all of the answers were true. (Always confirm your yes answers.)

- Start asking your specific, clear, and concise questions one by one. Confirm all yes answers by asking if that answer is correct. This ensures you are not tricking yourself and moving the pendulum for the answer you want.

When you get a No: When you get a no answer, you have a new series of questions to ask.

- "Is this spell harmful to me?"

- "Is this the wrong spell to cast?"

- "Is there something missing from my spell?"

- "Is there something I need to remove from my spell?"

- "Is there a better resolution to my problem?"

- "Would this backfire on me?"

Ask specific questions that will point you in the right direction. If the pendulum swings really hard in the no movement, it's a big no. Ask, "Do I need to stop moving in this direction?"

Closing the reading: Make sure you've gotten everything. Ask if there is anything else you need to ask about your spell. If not, then ask if the reading can be closed. If the answer is no, keep asking specific questions. Take a break if you need to—rest after question groups. Even weight lifters take a three-minute rest between sets.

If you can't close the reading, ask if you need to move to a more interpretive oracle and ask if you can interpret it yourself. Record all answers in your Candle Magic Journal. Note any changes you need to make to your intention, initial need, etc. Check before and after you set up your spell ingredients to see if anything major has changed. Regular use of your pendulum will make this a quick and easy process.

COIN DIVINATION—HEADS I WIN, TALES I WIN

The penny is one of my favorite magical items. You can use it to charge up any spell, and you can use it to divine whether your spell is the one you need. Don't stop with just spells, though: you can use the penny for any decision you are making with a flip of the coin. There is a state of chance when a coin is in the air that is susceptible to an energetic push. Where that push is coming from depends on how you set up the initial coin toss. Inviting in divine or ancestral influences takes the coin toss from random to a divination technique.

Divination with coins can be done with one, three, four, or five coins. Heads is a positive answer and tails is a negative answer, but the *number* of heads and tails can tell a story. The more coins you use, the more depth you can get on the answer. Still, there is a certain clarity that can come from a single coin flip. As simple as this system is, like the pendulum, setting up energetically, crafting your questions, and confirming the results can lead to very in-depth answers.

A one-coin toss leaves no room for interpretation. Heads = yes. Tails = no. This is handy when one coin is all you have or you are thinking too deeply and confusing yourself with other divination methods.

A three-coin toss gives you more options for answers, and there is power in the number three. You have two definitive answers and two maybe answers that lean in each direction. This is a good option if the number three means a lot to you or the spirit allies you work with.

A four-coin toss is used in Santeria and as a Hermes divination system and has five possible answers. In Santeria, fresh coconut pieces are used with the white side being heads and the brown side being tails. I personally use

Tip from your Aunt Jacki: When I first started building my magical candle recipes, I would use the pendulum over my recipe cards to see if every ingredient was in agreement. I would also use the pendulum to make sure the blessing and ingredients aligned correctly. This taught me how to read the subtle energies of each blend as I created them. Over time, I could feel when recipes were not jiving. When I no longer needed my pendulum, it magically disappeared from the special box I kept it in.

these definitions in the four-coin toss system as they are definite and give you clear direction.

The five-coin system has a spectrum of six possible answers from definitely yes to definitely no. There is room for interpretation and actually a lot of wiggle room to confuse or put in your own interpretation based on the outcome you really want. If you use the five-coin system, I recommend you take the time to flesh out the definitions for yourself and communicate with your spirits on what the answers truly mean.

Preparing the questions: Be specific, clear, and concise and ask only one short question at a time. Just like with the pendulum, ask only yes or no questions. The best questions are under ten words long. If you have a rambling question, you are confusing the situation and I'll bet you a coin flip you have two questions mashed into one. Review the examples in the pendulum directions for additional instructions.

Preparing to toss: You are divining messages from a higher realm, so prepare a space worthy of this divine guidance. Casting in front of your altar is highly recommended. You can sit at a table or use the floor. If you are going to use the floor, clean it up and lay a blessed cloth down. Many toss while standing up, but realistically, from this height, things bounce. Kneel, sit, or at the very least bend over to toss closer to the ground. Shake the coins in your hands vigorously and gently open up your hands, letting the coins fall. You are not really flipping or tossing, but dropping the coins.

Opening up for your reading: Take several calming breaths and use your favorite grounding technique to get centered. Invite your higher self and guides to talk to you through the flip of the coins. Ask your guides if they will talk to you through this coin toss reading. Toss your coins, and if you get an answer that is on the no side of the spectrum, do not continue in this method.

Asking the questions: Start with a prayer of gratitude for your spirit allies, ancestors, and guardians for guiding and protecting you. Invite your higher self and gatekeeper spirit to send the answers for your questions through the coins. Start by getting permission to do the reading.

It's like asking your friend if it's a good time to talk when you call out of the blue.

1. Ask if your higher self is ready and willing to answer your questions with truth and in your highest good.

2. Ask if your gatekeeper/guardian is able to keep out any negative or dishonest influences.

3. **If you get a yes** on all these questions, ask if all of the answers were true.

4. Start asking your specific, clear, and concise questions one by one. Confirm all yes answers by asking if the answer you got was true and in your highest good.

5. **If you get a no,** you have a new series of questions to ask.

   - "Is this spell harmful to me?"

   - "Is this the wrong spell to cast?"

   - "Is there something missing from my spell?"

   - "Is there something I need to remove from my spell?"

   - "Is there a better resolution to my problem?"

   - "Would this backfire on me?"

Interpreting your answers: The number of coins you toss will give you a different variety of answers. With any number of coins, if you get three or more no answers in a row, it may be time to close the reading.

One-Coin Toss

- Heads = Simple Yes

- Tails = Simple No

Three-Coin Toss

- 3 Heads = Strong Yes

- 2 Heads + 1 Tails = OK Yes

- 1 Heads + 2 Tails = Maybe Not

- 3 Tails = Strong No

Four-Coin Toss

- 4 Heads = Yes with peace and serenity but not necessarily blessings from spirit

- 3 Heads + 1 Tails = Ask again and clarify your question

- 2 Heads + 2 Tails = Absolutely yes, positive outcome with blessings from spirit

- 1 Head + 3 Tails = No—may have a negative outcome or an outcome that is not great

- 4 Tails = No, no, no. Extremely negative. Do not proceed.

Five-Coin Toss

- 5 Heads = Absolutely Yes!

- 4 Heads + 1 Tails = Strong Yes

- 3 Heads + 2 Tails = Cautious Yes

- 2 Heads + 3 Tails = Cautious No

- 1 Heads + 4 Tails = Strong No

- 5 Tails = Absolutely Not!

Closing the reading: It is crucial to close your reading as it is very disrespectful to your spirits if you don't. When you ask your friend if it's a good time to talk, you don't walk away or hang up without saying goodbye. When you are complete with your questions, ask if there is anything else you need to ask about your spell. If the answer is no, ask if the reading can be closed. If the answer to your "anything else" question is yes, keep asking specific questions until you get a no, and then ask if the reading is complete. If you cannot close the reading, ask if you need to move to a more interpretive oracle and ask if you can interpret it yourself.

Record all answers in your Candle Magic Journal. Note any changes you need to make to your intention, deeper need, etc. Check before and after you set up your spell ingredients to see if anything major has changed.

DICE—TAKING THE CHANCE OUT OF MAGIC

"It's the roll of the dice"—this is what we say when we are taking a chance on something with an outcome we can't easily influence. The symbol of dice in modern culture invites Lady Luck to the party: "Hello, Lucky 7!" Divining with dice flips the script and helps bring certainty and clarity where there was none. The system of divining with dice is very personal—there is little agreement from the experts. The number of dice can be from one to five, and the interpretations are read left to right with a combination of numbers or adding all the numbers together and then condensing them like you do in numerology. For instance: a dice roll gives you a 6 and a 5. 6 + 5 = 11. Condense 11 to 1 + 1 = 2.

Tip from your Aunt Jacki: If you take the dice from the Yahtzee game, don't put them back. Fully cleanse the dice you are pilfering and get a new set for the game. The last thing you want is Yahtzee becoming a source for divine communication. People get too serious, there ends up being a lot of crying, and you may get banned from future games.

I am utterly fascinated with dice as divination. There are so many dice divination systems on Etsy with three- to twelve-sided dice. That's a long way from the prehistoric throwing knucklebones as a way to cast lots. For checking in on your candle magic spell, I am going to keep it simple with a pair of dice for yes and no and the common interpretations from numerology. Once you use dice for divination, don't use them for anything else. Allow yourself to have divine objects that bring you powerful insight and truth. Just like any tool, the more people touch your divination tool, the more their energy will influence and skew the results.

Similar to the setup and opening in the coin divination, you will want a clean and blessed place to roll the dice. Use a cloth or a surface that won't cause them to bounce. Draw or mark a twelve-inch circle where the dice will land. If any land outside of the circle, do not include them in your reading.

Prepare your questions for yes and no answers, and invite in your divine allies and spirit guides. Get calm, grounded, and centered, then throw the dice, asking for permission to continue with the reading. (You can review the pendulum instructions for detailed steps.) When using yes and no divination tools, always double-check on your yes answers. Once you get the go-ahead, ask your question and throw the dice.

Interpreting the dice for yes and no questions: Odds are no. Evens are yes. If you are using two dice, add up the numbers to get your answer. (If you are using three or four dice, you can use the interpretations for heads and tails in the coin toss with even numbers representing heads and odd numbers representing tails.)

Interpreting the dice based on the numbers: A minimum of two dice are needed for this divination technique, as you need the possibility of adding the dice up to a nine. The interpretations are not an easy yes or no as some odds are a positive answer and some evens are a no answer. Throw your dice and add up the numbers until they condense down to a single digit. For example: You roll three dice and get a 5, 6, and 3. 5 + 6 + 3 = 14. Condense one more time. 1 + 4 = 5. Use the number 5 to interpret your answer.

Here are the basic numerological interpretations for this type of dice divination:

1: Your opinion is the driver in this spell. You have strong opinions and want to control all aspects of the outcome. If you have taken this spell from a book, stop and make it your own. There is something that you already feel isn't right or complete. Relax and get out of your head and into your heart to process your emotions before you cast this spell. Your candle spell will be successful if you do this.

2: Check your story. Your intuition about the spell you are casting is being influenced by your emotions. You may be creating a story around the situation that lives only in your imagination. Before you cast your spell, take inventory on what is the truth and what is an assumption. Do a spell for clarity and balance first or you will end up learning an uncomfortable life lesson.

3: Investigate your spell or the situation a bit further. There is either more that you need to include in the spell or the situation is bigger than you first thought. Find your joy within this spell and make sure you express it fully in the spell you crafted, as that is the driver for your success. If you move forward as is with your candle magic, you will not be as successful as you could be.

4 : You've got this. Do this spell as is because not doing it would land you in a worse situation. Let your intuition be your guide; it is spot-on. If this is a money spell, it will be very successful and help build a solid foundation. Getting the number 4 also tells you that you are going to have to do a bit of work in the physical world to achieve all the possibilities you woke up with this candle spell.

5: There is a big lesson for you in this spell. Ask more questions to get clarity on the outcome. Be curious as to why you want this spell; ask if this is the best option. Ask if there is anything to add or take away. Do not use a prewritten spell, but step into the freedom of crafting your own based on your unique need. Ask if you need to use another method of divination to get clarity, specifically the "Why Is That?" tarot reading.

6: Your spell will affect you internally before it affects your external world, helping you make peace with the inner struggle inspiring this spell. If this is a money spell, it won't go so well. If this is a relationship, family, or community spell, it will put you in a place of being the caregiver of the relationship or leader of the community. If this isn't what you want, start with a cord-cutting spell to ensure you are not manifesting someone else's idea of who you are.

7: Get quiet and listen to your intuition and psychic senses before casting this spell. The charm or blessing you write is very important; choose your words carefully. The results of the spell will be a mystery to you unless you look at it through a psychic lens. You may not see the results in the physical world right away as it needs to make its way through many people to get the outcome you want.

8: Your spell will have a slow start, but will end very successfully. This will be an example of your ability to create the world you want. Pay attention to what you did and how it goes. You will use this spell to remind you that magic is real. This spell will bring blessings to many. Get an additional boost to your spell by calling in your ancestors.

9: This is a very emotional spell for you, and you are asking for a big change or concluding a long life lesson. This spell will bring you deep wisdom and understanding. If you are doing a spell for material gain, it will come to you easily. Any spell you are doing will be successful if you keep what you are doing and the results to yourself so others cannot energetically interfere with it.

Don't forget to close! When you are done with asking questions, return to the yes and no method and ask if your reading is complete. If the answer is yes, thank your divine allies and move on to the next thing you are going to do. If the answer is no, keep asking questions as outlined in closing a coin toss reading.

Whatever method you use, check with the higher sources of wisdom before you do a spell that may cause more trouble than you are already in.

Tip from your Aunt Jacki: Mix it up! For fun I started using the dice to answer the positions in the Repercussions Tarot Spread and threw three dice for each of the four questions. Try this after you do your tarot spread. It will be spot-on each time and give a bit more clarity. Try them out as soon as you can pilfer your grandpa's Yahtzee dice.

THE JOY OF
SPELLCRAFTING

Put on your best Bob Ross because it's time to become a spellcraft-ing artist. The artistry in building a spell is not only undersung; spellcrafting has been turned into a stressful worry about getting everything *exactly right*. That's not how this works. Spells you find in books, online, or even prescribed to you by other practitioners are a *guideline* or *jumping-off point*. When you analyze the ingredients, words, timing of a predefined spell, you get to peek under the curtain of what makes that spell successful, but when you add your personality to it, your vision of success, and your own unique perspective, you have the power to do big magic. Your own "happy little accidents" are what allow spirit to fine-tune the vibration and make it stronger.

If you've ever watched Bob Ross on *The Joy of Painting*, you've see him start with a blank canvas and an intention for the type of landscape he is painting. He creates his palette of colors, sketches out the terrain, and builds the image stroke by stroke. Any one of those strokes makes no sense and looks like a blob of nothingness until they connect. When he makes a mistake, there is no eraser: there is only transforming that "happy little accident" into an interesting element in the larger picture. Ross is no Rembrandt—but he was never trying to be. *The Joy of Painting* was transformative during its time on air because it made artistry approachable and attainable just for the joy of doing so.

You are not Professor McGonagall, transmuting a prune into a rosebush; you are Molly Weasley tidying up your home and protecting your children. Your candle spell is all about creating an easier, better, and more joyful life for yourself. If you approach your spell with the exacting expectations of a great master, the fun will be replaced with fear of failure and self-doubt. If you approach your spell with the joy of stepping into magic for magic's sake and connection to the creative forces in the universe, you will be filled with possibilities and belief.

The ideas in this section are here to inspire your candle spell artistry to go beyond the match and wick and transform a candle spell into an experience that ignites your magic on every level—spirit, mind, emotion, and body. I will say this over and over again: you really can't get this wrong. You can take your magic on a different path, you can create something you were not expecting, you can doubt your spell into extinction—but you can't get it wrong. There are no wrong answers; there is only the experience that you are building. Build your spell with clear intent and then *pay attention* to the outcome. And there is *always* an outcome.

Right about now, there are magical folks that are falling out of their chairs screaming at this book: "*What do you mean you can't get it wrong!!*" If you take the Bob Ross approach to your magic and cocreate with your divine allies, you will begin a journey of discovery, balance, and awakening. Some outcomes will be as impactful as mild cheese, and some outcomes will be like a category four twister rampaging through your life—but neither outcome is *wrong* if that's the amount of energy needed to manifest your intent. If you are specifically going against your values and self-interest or stepping into someone else's lane, that is not intentional spellcrafting, that is something else entirely . . .

Tip from your Aunt Jacki: Magic works best as a growth process rather than a "get powerful quick" scheme. Calling on spirits that you have not built a loving relationship with, stealing someone else's power, or becoming judge and jury by cursing someone all qualify as jumping the gun and acting against your better nature. When you act outside of your nature, you are building up for a big backlash. Eventually, this negative energy becomes unsustainable and will come crashing down. That is, officially, getting it wrong.

HOW TO CHOOSE YOUR CANDLE

Did you do your "Why Is That?" exercise? It's OK if you already know what you need and want to fast-forward through this book. You will, however, still want to identify the branch or branches of magic you will be working your spell in. Knowing what type of magic will help you craft your best spell.

Your candle choice can be a pivotal point in building your spell. The style candle you choose to light will influence all the rest. Your candle choice may also be driven by what is available in the moment. Many times I have been inspired in the moment or needed to craft a spell on a holiday with no stores open. I looked around and used what was at hand and crafted the spell around that. Review how the different candles influence a spell and see where inspiration hits you.

CANDLE STYLES

Blessed and Dressed Candles

This is where my journey to becoming a candle magic expert began thirty years ago. I tried to prebless and dress a series of seven-day prayer candles, and instead of a magical experience, I had cracking and exploding glass from the flames shooting out of the top. I didn't know that oil-soaked kitchen string and a large handful of herbs would cause a brush fire on the top of my candles. I never thought that crystals could explode from the heat, either!

Back in the early 1990s candle-making supplies were not available at the local Michaels craft store, but I was determined to make my own blessed and dressed candle for efficiency's sake (and I had big ideas). After much experimentation and sound advice from the local candle-making supplier, I started pouring magical candles for a living. My Coventry Creations business literally came into being on my stovetop. I gave candles as gifts, and people wanted more. I was really surprised: why would people want one of my early awkward, ill-burning candles if they could dress and bless their own candles?

Why wouldn't they anoint their own and build their own spell? Over the past three decades I have lovingly discovered why some candle magic practitioners choose a dressed and blessed candle rather than doing it themselves:

1. The initial work is done for them, so it's a fast track to magic.

2. There are a lot of choices to make in creating your own candle spell and a premade one takes a lot of the guesswork out.

3. Some folks don't have the confidence to create their own spell.

4. They like the energy and can add their own for a bigger magical hit.

5. They are new to candle magic, and this is the gateway to more magic.

6. They have no desire to dress and bless their own ever.

7. They don't want to study all the magical uses of herbs and oils; they just want a spell.

8. They don't have the time or inclination to make this kind of mess in their home.

Back in 1992 I started the national intentional/magic candle market by taking my Blessed Herbal candles to stores in different parts of the country. Detroit, Seattle, Chicago, and Cleveland were the first stops on my journey. This was a new idea to every store I visited, and they were excited to get them. Within two years there were other companies cropping up to do the same thing I was. I had proven the market existed for this style of candle magic and inspired many variations on my initial theme. There are millions of people doing candle magic in one form or another now, and there is room for the many blessed and dressed candlemakers out there.

From Coventry to the small crafters on Etsy and everyone in between, magic candles abound and vary widely. Pillars, container candles, votives, tealights, and predressed seven-day candles—there is a style for everyone. Blessed candles have a magical efficiency to them, yet there is still room to add your own flair. You can add that with herbs, oils, curios, stones, and sigils that fine-tune the vibration of the candle to your unique intent. The colors, herbs, and oils of a blessed candle give you a running start to your candle spell, and then you can take the authority and add your own energy and magic.

Some makers, like Coventry, set up a mindful, magical workspace and charge up the candles with extra energy for you to use in your spell. I have purchased a few from other candlemakers because they felt amazing. Sometimes I need a different vibration to move past or uncover my energetic deficiencies, and a different magical candle helps me break through. If you choose a blessed or dressed candle, enjoy the vibe that was created for you.

The candles with the flowers, herbs, curios, and crystals embedded in them are so beautiful but require caution when burning. Please be aware that those herbs can flame up, the crystals can explode from the heat, and the curios can get hot and crack the glass (and/or burn your fingers when you pull them out). Stay attentive to any bedazzled candle you light. When the wax starts to melt, use tweezers or pliers to pull out anything that is embedded in the wax. It will not disrupt the magic. Think of it as the prize inside and place the item on your altar around the candle. The energy is still connected and active and now you can enjoy it in a safer way.

Remember to remove all packaging from your blessed and dressed pillar candles and place them in a candleholder. All container candles and candleholders can get hot at the bottom, so the best practice is to use an extra layer—like an upside down plate—between the candle and any surface that is easily marred.

Pillars, Tapers, and Votives

Pillars are stand-alone candles that you take all packaging off of. (Seriously, take all packaging off your candle before lighting it.) I like to call these naked candles "ready for magic." They come in a variety of sizes and are either paraffin or beeswax. Generally pillar candles don't drip a lot, but never assume they will ever be drip-free. Once you use a candle for a spell, your energetic need will change how the candle burns, potentially causing it to burn faster and drip more.

Tapers are the skinny candles that you see in old Dracula movies in the fancy candelabras. They are very popular on dining tables and can be very romantic. They are the original timekeepers and are wonderful in spells that are progressive and move step-by-step. For instance, you can place a pin or nail in the side of a taper candle when meditating, and when it falls, it makes a gentle sound to bring you out of a meditation.

Votive candles are a church specialty. The word *votive* comes from the Latin *votum*, meaning "vow" and *votivus*, meaning "promised by a vow."

When you go to a church to light a candle and say a prayer, you are making a vow before God. When you light a candle and say a prayer for someone living or dead, you are vowing your devotion to God, Jesus, or the Blessed Mother. So votives are for a single prayer, single purpose/vow that is said and released. Votives traditionally melt fast, requiring a candleholder to extend their burn time. Votives in a holder will have a ten- to eighteen-hour burn time depending on size.

A votive can also be used to recharge or rebalance a spell. One old-school practice uses a votive candle as a daily devotion for a long-term spell. The Catholic mothers that go to church to light a candle will go daily until that prayer is received and the issue resolved. They know that repetition is part of their prayer's success.

Chime candles are named for the Christmas angel chimes or *angel-abras*. The heat of the flame makes the delicate metal angels spin, hitting the small bell to create a chime sound. "The candles burn, the angels turn." Larger than a birthday candle, but smaller than a utility candle, with a two-hour burn time, chime candles are the perfect quick spell. They come in a rainbow of colors and are very inexpensive. These are great for recharging a spell, as a tool for refocusing, or as a series in a multiday spell. Just like votives, don't expect a huge result from one chime candle. If this is part of a big spell with a big ask, you will need to light many chime candles over time to keep the spell rolling.

Utility candles, also called sabbath candles, vigil candles, and emergency candles, are generally less than one inch in diameter and between four and seven inches high. They will burn for two to six hours depending on the size. These are white and you often see them used at candlelight vigils with the paper ring at the bottom to catch the drips. Utility candles are great altar offerings, quick spells, and they lend energy to non-candle spells. (Why would anyone ever do a non-candle spell?) They are excellent in cleansing work. I have the client hold a lit candle in each hand as I clear them and then wave them out when I am done to close the ritual.

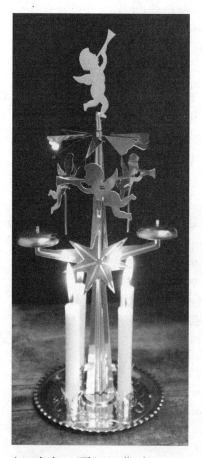

Angel-abra: "The candles burn, the angels turn."

THE BIG BOOK OF CANDLE MAGIC

Novena Prayer, Seven-Day, and Other Container Candles

Novena prayer candles are used in a Catholic ritual that lasts nine days. Novenas are prayed at the same time every day for those nine days and have a specific request of purpose. The Catholic Church discourages superstition and does not promise a miracle at the end of the nine days, yet there are many who receive the blessing they are asking for. Novenas are used for mourning, in preparation for a feast day, in penance, and to ask for God's intercession and a sign of his blessing.

Seven-day candles have inspired millions of candle spells over the almost century they have been in use. There is no definitive history of the seven-day candle, but it is reported that in the early 1940s Peter Doan Reed of the Reed candle factory in San Antonio, Texas, was the first candlemaker to produce the tall glass-encased candles with pictures of spiritual figures and an accompanying prayer. They are called seven-day candles because they burn continuously for about that amount of time and were based on the novena prayer candles found in Catholic churches. Where a novena is required to be said in the church, a seven-day candle can be burned at home as a daily ritual of giving thanks and asking for divine intercession.

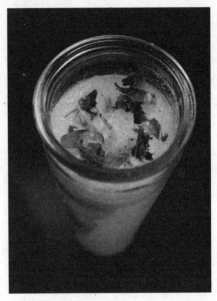

Stones, herbs, and glitter for a seven-day glamour spell.

Around the early 1970s Lama Temple Products out of Chicago started making more conjure-style seven-day candles. They screen printed the original spiritual figures and added candles such as 7 African Powers, Come to Me, Fast Cash, D.U.M.E., and many of the classics we still see today in botanicas and spiritual supply stores.

I started my own candle magic journey with the seven-day style of candles. I loved dressing them with herbs, oils, glitter, and images and turning the entire process into a ritual. I moved away from the seven-day candles into my own blessed candles, yet I return to them when I need their unique style. Seven-day candles are your go-to if you want to work with images, plan on working a vigil for a long time, or need to use the glass in other ways. Their purpose is highly driven by their color, with the white seven-day candles being an all-purpose choice.

Container candles are currently the most popular and easily accessible style of candles on the market as of 2022. They are self-contained, need no additional candleholder, and come in a variety of scents. Most container candles are white with a single or simple scent, making them mutable to your magical need. Just like the plain pillar candles, these are magic ready. You can dress them yourself, add images onto the glass, and treat them as a pillar/seven-day hybrid.

Figure Candles

Figure candles bring a whole different feel to your candle spell. They are so fun to work with, and in many ways it reminds me of when I was a child and the dramatic stories I would create and resolve with my Barbies. The symbology of the figure is a powerful foundation for the rest of your spell, and these are easy to dress with herbs, oils, and symbols. While there are the many shapes and styles available on the market today, I am focusing on the more traditional figure candles. You will find specific ways to dress these figures and other candles in the chapter "Prepping Your Candle for Magic."

Seven-Knob Candle

This is a seven-day spell candle, also known as a wish candle. It is not for a continual burn of the candle; you burn one knob every day for seven days. Use this candle when you have a big issue to work through that involves steps. Some examples are clearing debt bill by bill, getting through a competition, getting a mortgage, finding love.

You would make a wish on each knob of the candle, bringing what you want closer and closer to you until it manifests in full. Carve a wish on each knob of the candle, anoint it with oils and herbs that align with your goal, and/or place an anointed pin in each knob to fall away when that part of the spell manifests.

Cat

Why a cat? Cats have been associated with magic for centuries. They are said to have nine lives and always land on their feet. They are amazing hunters and never go hungry in the wild. Cats can get in and out of seemingly secure places (except for Schrödinger's cat, that poor thing has been in a box forever). Cats are very lucky, and a cat candle can be used to bring luck, second chances, and to hunt and catch things that seem elusive or out of your reach. Use a cat candle to work with your cat familiar or cat spirit and energy to foster communication. You can also use a black cat candle to steal the luck of another.

Cross

This candle is easily used as an altar piece to pray for a specific outcome and to gain the blessing of Jesus and the saints in any work you do. Anointed, the cross candle can be used for divine protection in any situation. If you are working to heighten your Christ consciousness, the cross candle is an excellent asset. Paired with crossed keys, the cross candle is also used as a representation of your own personal crossroads or clearing a crossed condition.

Devil

Candles in the shape of a devil are mainly used for banishing evil and negativity. Of course, they can also be used to curse. In the Christian cosmology, the devil and his minions are the cause of all suffering, pain, and violence; thus using a devil candle in a Run Devil Run spell will drive that influence out of your life.

The devil candle is also used to bring a cornucopia of earthly delights. As the fallen angel who has dominion over earth, you can use the devil candle to bring money, love, power, and anything that is associated with your earthly life. You can bedevil someone, manifesting the trickster to get your way or beat the odds. The horned gods of old were often labeled as minions of the devil, making this a candle that will assist in calling to their earthly, primal power or the trickster and party gods that also are horned.

Tip from your Aunt Jacki: Run Devil Run is an old conjure spell with its root in Mexican curandero folk healing. This spell is similar to uncrossing with the addition of a "Not today, Satan" vibe. If uncrossing is not working for you, Run Devil Run is the next level of intensity. Run Devil Run or "Corre Diablo Corre" will banish bothersome entities, clear away negative intent that has been directed at you, and even help you clear out your own destructive tendencies. I use this spell when I am dealing with my own personal demons and find I am falling down a well of despair.

Human Figure Candles

Whatever you are thinking right now about what a human figure candle represents, you are correct— they can be used for lust spells. It's painfully apparent that these candles are used to represent someone and bring focus to a spell that involves a specific person.

They are also wonderful for manifesting someone that is yet to be named. Human figure candles are very effective in moving spells where you are drawing someone to you or sending them away.

Obviously use the female or male figure candle as appropriate to the person's gender. If your target is gender-fluid, you can use the gender candle they are most closely associated with, or change the physical appearance of the candle to be sexless.

The purpose of the spell is often directed by the color of candle you use. Red for sex, pink for love, green for money, purple or white for healing, etc. When you dedicate the figure candle to a specific person, scribe their name on the bottom of the candle and place a name paper under the candle.

Genitalia

Now we are getting really specific. Genitalia candles are used almost exclusively for candle spells to draw a new lover to you, increase passion in a relationship, keep your partner faithful, or keep them captivated by you and your sexual relationship.

Yoni vulva candles are for drawing a female lover or for heating up a woman's own appeal as a female lover. You can also use this representation for woman power in candle spells that call to the bitch goddess within.

Phallus penis candles are also for drawing a male lover and for increasing a man's passion and sexual prowess. You can also balance a man's sexual energy depending on the color of the candle chosen; white and blue candles cool a man's sexual appetite, while red and purple will increase it.

Lovers

This candle is for passion—starting it or stoking it. The lovers are for an existing romantic relationship and igniting passion, reconciling, fertility, building friendship, clearing outside influence, etc. You can use this in place of a marriage candle if needed. You can also create your own lovers combination by connecting genitalia candles.

Marriage

The figure candle that looks like a wedding cake topper is used specifically for marriage—to bless it, inspire it, heal it, or break it up. Where the lovers candle is more about the sexual relationship, the marriage candle is more about the overall relationship. The two can be employed for each other in a pinch.

You can also create your own marriage candle by connecting two figure candles with a string or cord or heating them up so they stick together.

Skull

The skull candle is for working with the mind or with spirits that were once human. They are used in healing spells to connect with the whole spirit, higher self, or root of the issue. Most descriptions of skull-candle use center on connecting to another's mind to read it, confuse it, or influence it. If this is your goal, having a personal concern or a detailed name paper is required for the spell to be successful. My favorite way to use the skulls is to create cooperation between two people and to influence your own mindset.

Skull candles are very popular for working with ancestors and helpful spirits. You can use the skull as the focal point in your altar by carving in the name of the spirit or ancestor and anointing it with herbs and oils.

Pyramid

Pyramid candles are for manifestation. The shape of a pyramid is considered magical in most traditions as it grounds, focuses, and increases the power of the intent. Books have been written just on this shape and the energy it generates by its presence. The US dollar has a pyramid on it, adding divine power and blessing to the currency. You would not go amiss by adding a pyramid candle to any manifesting spells as it brings power to your intention and speed to the final manifestation. A well-phrased intention and words of power inscribed on a pyramid candle are powerful all on their own.

SIZE

Size matters! Matching your need to the right size of candle saves your patience in both directions. If you have a simple, quick spell and choose a long-burning candle, you are either wasting three-quarters of the candle or waiting forever for it to be done. If you have a big spell and use a chime or votive candle, you may be waiting for the results that don't come because you shortchanged your spell.

Think about what you are doing and how big of a change it is. The bigger the magical task, the more personal attention and ritual your candle spell will need to be successful. If you think you can use one votive or chime candle for a big spell and get the results of a larger candle, be ready for disappointment.

When customers ask me if they can "just use a votive, it is less expensive" for a money-drawing spell, for instance, I ask them if they want to find a new good-paying job or five dollars dropped in the street.

I can never say this too much: *Never leave a burning candle unattended!* Fire is wild and unpredictable, especially when you add the vibration of magic to it.

Long-burning candles, seven-day candles, or large pillars are your choice for spells that will take time to manifest or as an altar candle for an ongoing spell. You can even dedicate a large candle to a specific issue that comes up frequently. You will be attending that candle every day, if not several times a day, to renew your intention and keep the magic moving. Large pillars need a large candleholder. Don't risk an unprotected candle: fire is unpredictable and I have seen it jump in the weirdest ways.

Figure candles and medium-sized pillar candles are your choice for a specific spell. Figure candles burn faster and need a platter to burn on and continual attention. The less-expensive figure candles don't always have a straight wick and things can literally go sideways on you. Medium-sized pillar candles, depending on burn time, can also have a surprising burn style and need to be attended while burning. These midsize candles are good for moving spells where you will be changing the position of the candle throughout your spell. Remember to use a candleholder for every pillar and make sure it is large enough to hold all the wax of the candle. When you add energy to any candle, it becomes unpredictable. Because I never leave a burning candle unattended, my midsize candles often last several days.

Votive, chime, and tealight candles are for your quick spell, a burst of energy for an ongoing spell, or to be used sequentially over a period of time to build up energy. I do like tealight and chime candles for meditation timekeepers. If I am working with my prosperity altar and am doing a gratitude practice, I will light an anointed tealight for that particular moment. On my overall magic altar, if I see there is a struggle for the day—whether astrologically or in real life—I will grab a votive to counter that energy and let it burn all day.

TYPE OF WAX

You may have heard that soy wax is less toxic and paraffin is from the devil. The soy-wax industry must have an amazing PR department. I have been making candles for thirty years, and when I started, soy wax was not a thing.

My choice was between paraffin and beeswax, and with the price and availability of beeswax, paraffin was clearly the only sustainable choice for my candles. When the initial reports on soy wax came out in the early 2000s, I was terrified I was doing something horrible to the environment and researched all of my wax choices. Not all wax is equal, and there are different uses and specialties, it's true. But I stayed with paraffin and am proud to help keep 156 tons of wax per year from being dumped in various places.

Paraffin is a by-product of the oil industry. It is created when they purify crude oil into petrol. It is used in pillars, votives, tealights, and some container candles. Up until the early 1990s, oil companies would pay to have paraffin taken away, and what wasn't used in industries was dumped. There are grades of paraffin that are used by different industries, with the highest grade (least amount of crude oil in the wax) employed in the medical and food industries. The harder the wax, the less crude oil it contains. Pillar candles are made from a higher-grade wax than is used in the adhesives, coatings, or rubber industries.

Beeswax is a naturally occurring wax that is used in pillars, votives, and tealights. It was the primary wax used for candles throughout history. It is harder than paraffin and burns at a higher temperature. There is a lovely smell to natural beeswax, which will influence any scent added to it. Beeswax is harvested by cutting the caps off of the cells in a beehive that holds the honey. They are then drained of all honey, frozen or chemically treated to get rid of moths and beetles, and then processed for use as a commercial wax. Not all beekeepers sell the wax; many keep it to set up the foundation of the next year's honey harvest.

Soy wax is made from soybean oil. It is a soft wax that must be put in a container candle. It is most often blended with other waxes—palm, paraffin, or bees—to improve its look, burn quality, and scent management. The soy industry has spent a lot of money scaring people away from paraffin, but soy is not as sustainable as it claims. There are concerns about pesticides and GMO issues that are causing an increasing number of allergies. Since soy requires a container, the fossil fuels burned to create and move those containers really just end up creating more paraffin.

Palm and other waxes are growing heroes in the candle industry and top-of-the-line expensive. Palm is one of the only natural waxes that can be used to make pillars, but it has to be blended with a harder wax or stearine additives that are animal and petroleum by-products. Palm wax comes from palm oil, and there are concerns with deforestation around the explosion of palm crops. Coconut and rapeseed waxes are newer to the market, and there is less information about them. Coconut wax is softer and used for container candles. It holds scent well and does burn fast. It is also the most expensive of all the waxes. Rapeseed wax is essentially a hardened vegetable oil and used in pillars and container candles.

When picking your candle, be wary of the hype of any wax being the ultimate amazing and perfect answer. Just because something says it is eco-friendly, organic, and sustainable doesn't mean it is. There is no regulation on packaging for this industry. Go with what works for you and your spell.

COLOR

Your first magical response is driven by color and your emotional resonance with it. Colors are your mood setter. Think about walking into a room painted in a color you don't vibe with where you already feel the disharmony and mood shift. Inversely, think about your current favorite color and your mood is elevated. Why?

In 1666 Sir Isaac Newton discovered the prism effect, where pure white light separates into visible colors. Since then, the study of color and its effect upon the world began. Wavelengths were measured, vibrations assigned, and sciences/therapies developed around them. Color psychology is a term in art, design, and marketing. There are books upon books cataloging colors, shades, and tone in emotional categories. Have you noticed that banks have moved from the authority of blue logos to the welcoming and sustainable energy of green? Color psychology dictates product design, ad placement, and anything that requires the approval of the masses.

In the world of magic, my philosophy is that colors have very strong vibrations that pull the vibration of other ingredients to match. If you are using a red candle and combine it with ingredients that have a subtle, gentle vibration, the red will influence the rest to be more in line with its aggressive, powerful nature.

Your emotional reaction to the color affects its vibration. Your response is influenced by the culture you are indoctrinated in and the value given to the color. The vibration of the color influences your energy, your reaction to the color influences its vibration, and this becomes a feedback loop that can grow stronger and stronger when you apply intent and magic to it.

In the Siddha yoga tradition there is a blue pearl that lives at the top of the crown chakra. This blue is said to illuminate the mind and everything beyond the body. When this blue color is brought into meditation, it can take you to new worlds. There is the feedback loop of that blue creating a response and the understanding of that blue increasing its vibration. This doesn't happen for me as I don't have that cultural connection and blue is not in my top five favorite colors.

As you choose your starting color for your spell, think about how you respond to that color. If you hate green to the core of your being, using it for prosperity is going to create a negative feedback loop that may short out your magic. (If you hate green, maybe it's time to think about why and how that affects your prosperity.)

The information in the Color Index is my take on the standard meaning of colors. You will see I deviate from what any online search results tell you. Right here is an example of how *you* make magic *your own* and how it is open to your personal interpretation. Just like the meaning of herbs, this is your jumping-off point to develop your own color mastery.

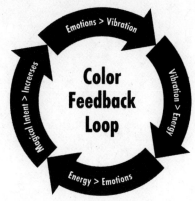

Does color feed our magic, or does our magic feed the color?

Ninety percent of the time, you pick your candle because it is available and easy. Any candle will do for any spell. You may have to adjust the spell to fit the resources, but that is a sign of a crafty witch. Work smart not hard. Everything can be substituted for something similar. As you master your candle magic, you will gravitate to one type of candle because it is easy and works for you. You may even dive into making your own candles—but that is another book for another time.

PREPPING YOUR CANDLE
FOR MAGIC

"Light and go" is a very acceptable way to do preblessed candle magic. That's what I do when I have a need and limited time. I grab my tranquility candle when I am going to an event with lots of people of differing opinions to help keep the peace. I light a prosperity candle when I am reconciling my bank accounts. I light a love's enchantment candle when I am preparing for date night with my husband. Then there are times, however, when I need to go full-on badass witch and get my ritual on. This is when I spend time creating my "Why Is That?" story and choosing all the parts and pieces that will go into that candle spell. I choose my herbs, colors, ritual time, and type of candle. Then I add in the accessories that make the spell personal to me and my needs. I let my why be my guide and use the right symbology to tell my tale to my magical self and the universe. Crafting this united energy makes my magic inevitable.

CHOOSING OILS AND HERBS

The magical boost you can get from herbs and oils is worth the time you will take to review what ingredients synchronize with your intent. If you are new to the magical herb world, step into your kitchen, scan your cooking herbs and spices, and start there. Between your spice rack and your yard, you have tons of magic at your fingertips.

Blending herbs and oils is my magical go-to. I love this part of creating my candle spell most of all. Calling in the devas (spirits) of the herbs and oils and connecting them to the spell I am creating make a larger, focused energy to feed my intent. When I first started blending herbs ages ago, I didn't realize what I was doing. I had just learned how to feel the energy of things, and I instinctively started combining my ingredients until I felt the energy and vibration that seemed connected to the intent I wanted. There was no system to it; I was working from a place of awe and trust in magic. I look back at the early days of my discoveries and reminisce over that freedom. I kind of miss when everything felt like a miracle; there was so much childlike innocence and I was excited over every new thing I learned. Now that I am a seasoned, jaded adult witch, I realize how much that sense of wonder adds to my magical practice.

In 2007, when I started teaching the Coventry Magic classes, I had the opportunity to reconnect with the herbs and oils in an intimate, wondrous way, and they didn't disappoint. With my experienced witch perspective, our relationship became richer, more seasoned, and again filled with awe. The brilliance of nature shows in the variations that every plant gives you and how each fills the world with a special vibration.

Clarification from your Aunt Jacki: For simplicity's sake, I am using the word *herb* to reference herbs, resins, barks, roots, spices, berries, oils, and all types of plant parts.

The power of the deva or spirit of nature within each herb is an amalgamation of all aspects of energy that come together to create that plant. For instance, the basil you use in your spaghetti sauce and love spell had to grow from a seed, fed by the nutrients in the soil, sun, and rain. The wind and insects pollinated it to expand and grow, increasing its energy. The deva or magic that grows within the basil is born from all the other spirits of nature that contributed to its existence, including what died and decomposed to feed the soil. The deva is always present no matter the source of your basil: growing, fresh-cut, infused, distilled, or dried for longevity—the magical spirit of that herb is just a whisper away. Dried herbs are often seen as dead and lacking energy, yet if you call to the deva of that plant with a whisper and an invitation from your heart, its energy can still blossom for magical use. Let's compare this to turning on the radio. When the radio is off, the waves that deliver the music are still in the air, but we can't hear them. When you turn on the radio (your psychic energy) and tune in to a station (the herb), you get the radio waves that carry the classic rock or what have you that you are looking for (the deva).

My first blends started with recipes I found in books, but I often disagreed with the details. They were often not right for me or the intent I was blending for. It wasn't that the author was wrong; it was not a competition. They gave me a basic idea, but I needed to reblend the spell for my own needs. Those recipes also gave me something to question. Why did Scott Cunningham create a House Wealth Incense with frankincense, myrrh, patchouli, allspice, nutmeg, and ginger? Why not cinnamon? Why not orange blossoms? Why use frankincense for prosperity when it's one of the best resins to use for an exorcism? How do those intersect? Is someone just making this stuff up?

As you dig into the uses of herbs, you master that magic of perspective. There is an energy and a vibration to each ingredient, and they can be used in many ways. Think about a crowbar. It can be used to leverage something heavy, pry up nails, create an opening, or become a weapon. It's the same shape, weight, and density for each one of those operations, but its uses are many. Now let's apply this idea to frankincense.

Frankincense is used for protection, cleansing, spirituality, meditation, anxiety, fear, obsessions, and exorcism. Why would it be in an incense for house wealth? Looking at the big picture and overall energy of frankincense, we can see it reduces stress. It has a powerful, high vibration that displaces negative energy with its own spiritual vibe. That in turn brings a sense of peace and connection with the divine. It sounds like good old Frank will clear the way for all the other ingredients to work their magic. It's hard to get spiritual when you are in a stressed state, making frankincense a resin that you can use for multiple purposes.

With so very many herbs and oils to work with, how do you get down to what is best for your spell? It's almost worse when your selection of herbs grows and you get into analysis paralysis for what you want for your spell. Remember less is more with your blends. Let your plant helpers shine their energy and collaborate with their fellow ingredients to complement and not compete. With more than five ingredients you run the risk of choosing ones that will cancel each other out. There is no quick table to tell you what cancels what; it is a very energetic experience. Use your tools—a pendulum works well here—with each addition, and check your progress along the way. Go slow and you will be rewarded.

If you are looking for a system to start with and learn from, this seasoned and salty witch has finally

Tip from your Aunt Jacki: I started my magical journey before the internet. Hidden wisdom had to be sought out in old herbal books and hunted down in any books on magic. The challenge of scouring used bookstores and finding the small spiritual shops in out-of-the-way places was part of the magic. I absorbed everything I could, reading cover to cover and understanding the bigger picture of what the author was going for. Now I can google a spell and compare site to site for what I am looking for. I find that many of us 21st-century magical practitioners are copying the same things over again and most of the recipes are from those old books I found. The same spell is on ten different sites with the exact same wording. Look at that spell, the ingredients, the symbology, and understand its "Why Is That?" This deconstruction of a spell will teach you more than ten hours of classes.

created one to help you build your herb and oil blend with minimal conflict. Try my process and, as you master it, develop your own system. I will not be offended by this divergence, and I would probably learn something from you. I'm not here to lay down dogma, but to inspire you and get you rolling with your magic.

In my Magical Herb Index, I focus on the most common options available at any spiritual, grocery, or health food store. Start with what you easily know, and as you master this process, go ahead and get exotic with your ingredients. Most are only an internet search away.

The Magic 5 Blends

Five points on the pentagram, five elements (including spirit), the symbol of a crossroad, the number of fingers and toes we have on each limb, the second easiest multiplication table to master, the number of levels in Maslow's hierarchy of needs, and the number of magical branches to manifesting what you need—five is a magic number. In each magical intent, addressing all five branches helps to attain your goal and evolve from it. Five ingredients is all you will ever need for a spell—one for each branch of magic. Building your spell to address all five levels of actualization and magic will manifest your goal faster.

Musings from your Aunt Jacki: You have to have fresh clean water to clean other things. Putting new socks in dirty water only creates dirty socks. Making sure you have clean energy in the space where you are working allows the magic to happen. Leaving the energy congested makes it harder for your work to bust through.

For instance, I did a spell to keep the words flowing out of my fingers and into my book. A simple creativity spell? Yes, and it needed to tune in to me. I am writing, not painting. I am writing from my experience, not creating a new story. I need to be very productive with my writing time because I am also running a wildly expanding business at the same time. My needs are different from the fiction writer or the portrait photographer, so my blend must meet *my* needs. My creativity blend will be built from my own personal why and will address each branch of magic and how it affects my intent.

Creative Flow Spell

Why is that? *I have a small window to write, and I need to stay focused and prolific.*

THE BIG BOOK OF CANDLE MAGIC

Why is that? *This book is really important to me to finish, and I am worried I don't have enough to say.*

Why is that? *This is a celebration of the candle magic I have been teaching for decades, and next year (2022) is the thirtieth anniversary of Coventry being in business.*

My "Why Is That?" brought me these keywords: confidence, abundance, focus, clarity, creativity, longevity, support, sabotage, flow, inner strength.

From these keywords, I could find my deficit and the ways that the Magic 5 can work together to give me the energy I need to bring my spell to life. What is my deficit? Calm confidence. How do I fill my deficit with the calm confidence I need to finish my book?

Healing: I need to heal the imposter belief.

Clearing: I need to clear the fears of others that could stop my progress.

Love/Relationships: I need the support of the people around me to create the space to write.

Protection: I need to protect myself and my business from sabotage.

Prosperity: I need to have the confidence that the money is flowing and I can focus on writing.

What herbal ingredients do I need to add to my spell candle to create this energetic focus?

Healing: Ginger to remind me of the power that I inherently hold inside. I am never an imposter. I am simultaneously an eternal student and master adept.

Clearing: Eucalyptus to uncross my energy and clear away the jealousy and hooks that others have laid in my path.

Love/Relationships: Basil to increase my confidence and create a cooperative relationship with the people around me. It elevates everyone's spirit and helps them see the big picture of this book and get excited.

Protection: Anise to keep the evil eye away and alert me to any incoming attack.

Prosperity: Cinnamon to raise my vibration, reminding me to trust in the processes I have created and keep communication channels open.

I chose these five powerful ingredients because their energies aligned and I had them handy and available. In my cupboard I have fresh ginger, dried basil, anise, and cinnamon. I have a muscle rub made from eucalyptus essential oil. As I added them into my bowl, I called the name of the ingredient, asked it to bring its specific power to a part of my spell, and invited it to be a part of my spell. When I was done blending, I was charged up and my face was red from the energy pull. Together the herbs and oil made a surprisingly lovely paste giving me something that will stick to the candle. I also had a Coventry Creations Lakshmi candle and several utility tealights to start this spell. Once I added my words of power and set up my temporary altar, my spell was active and powerful.

Even as I write about this spell, I feel the energy of it fill me again. It was *my* spell, *my* blend, and *my* success. Now, as I continue to write this book, I can call up that spell at any time to fill me with the boost from the deva I created with this blend of ingredients.

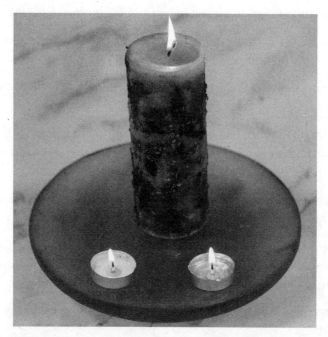

This is my Creative Flow Spell after a "Why Is That?" exercise.

THE BIG BOOK OF CANDLE MAGIC

Now it's your turn. Grab the "Why Is That?" worksheet you started in chapter one and look through your answers, keywords, and patterns. In your Candle Magic Journal, start to identify and write down the energetic and magical deficit for each of the Magic 5. Leave room to note the ingredients you want for each branch. It may be several herbs for each branch as you decide on the best ones for your spell from what is readily available to you.

Check out the herb and oil combinations below for inspiration and flip to the Magical Herb Index in the back of the book to scan for your unique needs. I made it easy and gave you how the herb works in each of the Magic 5. Relax, connect to the plant world, and let the answers you need come to you. Please, do not overthink this. Your ingredients will listen to you and do their energetic best. Close your eyes and think of the first word to float to the surface.

Example Herb and Oil Blends

My library is packed with magic herbal recipe books from the likes of Scott Cunningham, Paul Beyerl, Ray Malbrough, and Amy Blackthorn, to name but a few. These are all wise authors whose recipes are trustworthy and powerful. I have referenced them many times as I put together spells in the past. Between their books, information online, and the recipe ideas I have added to this book, I challenge you to ask powerful questions.

Why are those ingredients effective in those recipes?

How do the devas of each ingredient work with each other?

How will they work with my particular spell?

Are there any ingredients that can be or need to be swapped out?

When I see a question in my inbox of "This candle spell didn't work the way I wanted it to, now what?" I take my customer through a quick "Why Is That?" We discover what complications were not addressed with the chosen candle. The only thing wrong will always be a missing something that would fine-tune the energy to exactly what they needed. It could be a combination of candles and oils, an addition of herbs or stones, or even a bit of ritual. Most candle spells will get the spell done in one; it's when one misses the mark that digging in deeper is the better answer.

The following blend examples use the balance of the Magic 5 to address the energetic deficit that may be occurring with each unique magical need.

Use these as inspiration for your own blends or create them as is to explore how each interacts with your own needs.

Prosperity

Prosperity needs come in different flavors for many different energetic deficits. The blend for an immediate cash need is different from work issues. A blend to create long-term wealth is different from financial success. There are ingredient standards for prosperity spells. What you blend in conjunction with those standards is the art of fine-tuning the candle spell to your specific need. Let's have some fun!

Money-Drawing Spells

I Need Cash Now—Fast Cash Spell

> **Prosperity:** Cinnamon raises your vibrations, brings confidence, and is a general money-drawing herb. Money is attracted to those who vibrate confidence in its continual return.

> **Protection:** Myrrh expands your awareness on all levels. It too raises your vibrations to bring the peace, confidence, and balance needed to fortify your security. Myrrh is a favored partner of frankincense and together they create heaven on earth.

> **Love:** Patchouli connects you with the rhythm of life and attunes you to its flow. This is an excellent money herb, and through its calming nature, it attracts people who align with you and may give you money or support its creation.

> **Clearing:** Frankincense is another vibration-raising herb that clears your anxieties and fears. This will help you release your money worries and step into the confidence that patchouli and myrrh are creating.

> **Healing:** Sandalwood's high vibration pushes away any negativity that may be causing your dis-ease. It increases the power of any ingredient it is used with and awakens a sense of peace.

Thieves in the Temple—Recover Lost or Stolen Money Spell

> **Prosperity:** Lemongrass opens the road to new prospects of prosperity. It transforms any bad luck to good and prosperous energy.

Protection: Evergreen (pine) fortifies your strength and protects your home base from any additional loss.

Love: Dates bring in the sweetness of life and remind you that any setback is temporary.

Clearing: Orange blossom banishes the anxiety-ridden negative thoughts that would limit the return of what was lost.

Healing: Jasmine brings peace to your spirit and heals any karmic lessons, blocks, or self-sabotage that may have contributed to your loss.

Protection

Protection work is very personal and every situation has a different spin and need. When you are securing your safety, calm confidence is the cornerstone to your magical success. Yet it is hard to attain that state once an attack begins, because attacks are geared to create a chaotic disruption. All of my protection spells contain ingredients that will ground, center, and calm you within the swirl of chaos. Protection spells also need to be varied over time. Like the Borg in *Star Trek*, attacking energy will adapt in frequency over time and break through. In the examples below, replace the herbs as they pertain to your specific situation. Magic involves continual experimentation, so go have some fun!

Give Me Shelter from the Storm—Protection Spell

Prosperity: Geranium will protect family property and wealth from harm or loss.

Protection: Agrimony's superpower is protection from negativity in all its forms. It builds the foundation of your fortress of safety.

Love: Blessed thistle is aggressively protective and will keep unwanted attention away. It will also drive away people who intend to harm you in any way.

Confessions from your Aunt Jacki: I am a sci-fi nerd and many of my spells reflect their modern-day mythology. Today's supernaturals are found in the comics, movies, TV shows, and books. On the sci-fi nerd scale, I only rank a 5 or 6 so please don't quiz me, since I will fail the test of any nerd at a 7 or higher.

Clearing: Frankincense's high vibrations clear the fears and stressors that sap your energy. It in turn refills you with the purity and strength that come with divine protection.

Healing: Dragon's blood brings balance and harmony to your protection spell to keep it strong and flexible as your needs change. It also powers up all other ingredients in your spell.

Under Attack—Neutralize Attack, Sabotage, and/or Abuse Spells

Prosperity: Eucalyptus will clear away any attacks on your abundance or success. It will pull away the hooks and mental confusion sent your way to make you uncertain.

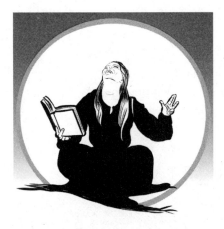

Evolve your protection spells as you evolve.

Protection: Tarragon protects women, children, and those who are at the mercy of their abusers. It helps them reclaim their strength and independence. It will bring clarity of mind and confidence in what you are really perceiving to be true.

Love: Allspice will refill your energy, boost your confidence, and make it easier to see who fills your life with love and support and who is sending negativity.

Clearing: Angelica brings in angelic protection that drives out hexes and curses. It is also protective of those who are at the mercy of their attackers, helping to clear out the mental confusion created by trauma.

Healing: Cayenne and chili peppers of all types will break hexes, set up a protective barrier, heat up your determination, and speed up your results.

Love

Love them or hate them, love spells are controversial. Are you compelling and manipulating someone with a love spell, or are you creating a vibration that makes the love match more likely? From my own perspective, magic works first on you before it moves out into the wider world. So when you are casting a healthy, balanced spell, you are first prepping yourself to receive the magic as it is manifesting. A love spell first works on you, helping to heal the deficiency or wound that has you seeking love in the first place. To find new love, you must feel lovable, or you will miss the signs when a new love shows up in your life. To deepen the love in a marriage, you must fall deeper in love too. Even self-serving love spells will teach you about your own fears, blocks, issues, and deficiencies, albeit this usually comes the hard way if you are not paying attention to the signs to heal.

Call Me Maybe—Come to Me Spell

A come to me spell has a specific person in mind when you are casting it. You are sending the message that you are definitely interested and ready for their attention. Come to Me will draw them to you, but it cannot make them love you. This is all about the initial pheromone chemistry that pulls someone in. Then it's up to you to land that fish by getting to know them, connecting where you are compatible, and encouraging love to grow.

Prosperity: Catnip will heat up your appeal and charm the one you are interested in. It helps you get lucky!

Protection: Cayenne will heat up the passion between you and protect from the influence or jealousy of others.

Love: Damiana will sway someone to your side and inspire interest and lust.

Clearing: Orange blossom clears you of nervousness and frigid behavior in matters of love.

Healing: Nutmeg builds confidence in your appeal and inspires your interest being returned to you.

Everybody Needs Somebody to Love—New Love Spell

Prosperity: Clove is a drawing spice that builds confidence and pulls new people into your orbit.

Protection: Lavender will draw new love to you while protecting you from anyone cruel or abusive.

Love: Jasmine warms your spirit, opening you to love and attracting that love and passion into your life.

Clearing: Peony helps you see the love that surrounds you. It also helps you be mentally and emotionally clear on the type of person you want to attract so you can focus on that passion and affection.

Healing: Aloe soothes the feelings of loneliness and brings divine support in finding your new love.

Clearing

Getting unstuck with a good clearing helps you manage your energy, especially when that energy is bogged down with every spirit and person you've crossed paths with. When this heaviness is lifted, life is easier, clearer, happier, and you get to be yourself without interference. Candle magic is effective for this magic as it will draw off the energy and consume it in the flame so that it cannot quickly return to you.

Break That Spell/Curse

Prosperity: Cinnamon clears the blocks to your prosperity and gets you to the other side of the stress so you can see and understand the cause of it.

Protection: Lemongrass transforms any negative energy into positive and breaks through the lies into the truth.

Love: Nettles will break through manipulation and crush the spell that was cast at you.

Clearing: Frankincense raises your vibration to the divine level and casts out a spell or curse directed at you.

Healing: Myrrh is the essence of the phoenix reborn. It burns away what limits and harms you and helps you break free of curses or hexing.

Blockbuster

Prosperity: Lemongrass opens the road to new ideas and transforms your doubts into certainties.

Protection: Cinnamon protects you from the influence of others and allows your mind to break free of its constraints.

Love: Orange blossom clears your fears around embracing all of your power. It invites cooperation and support from your loved ones.

Clearing: Ginger brings triple strength to your spell, pushing out anything that may attempt to block you.

Healing: Dragon's blood powers up any spell to a blockbuster level.

Healing

Magic = Healing and Healing = Magic. This is a core principle of the magical techniques I teach. When you are bringing magic into your life, you are creating energetic healing opportunities. When you heal your energy, this is an opportunity to create a magical change in your life. Healing magic supports a mastery of the arcane arts: psychic development, meditation, divination, and spellcrafting. It also supports your personal spiritual growth. Healing addresses the limitations that are within, where clearing addresses the limitations on the outside.

Hear My Inner Voice/Guardian Angel/Spirit Guides

Prosperity: Sage is very empowering, cleansing and helping you find your voice even when you are stressed.

Protection: Tarragon is very protective of you in oppressive situations. It brings you confidence and strength.

Love: Dandelion draws benevolent spirits and opens your mind and spirit to seeing who is surrounding you.

Clearing: Saffron breaks up oppressive energy so your inner light awakens and connects you with the divine.

Healing: Angelica fills you with an abundant amount of good, healing energy, lifting your vibrations up to communicate with your guardian angels.

Develop My Psychic Intuitions and Spirituality

Prosperity: Anise opens up your psychic centers, brings in divine influences, and helps you see the possibilities around you.

Protection: Aloe shares divine protection as you are opening and discovering your powers.

Love: Copal raises your vibration and clears out the expectations of the people around you, allowing you to see the bigger picture.

Clearing: Dandelion clears the psychic centers of confusion.

Healing: Parsley transcends this world and opens you up to understanding other dimensions. It creates a clear channel to the divine.

HOW TO DRESS AND BLESS

It's time to put your chosen herbs and oil to work in a safe way. You will be addressing a central contradiction in candle magic: candles are all about that flame, and herbs and oils are flammable. Working smart and safe means a little bit of herbs goes a long way, as too many dried herbs on your candle will create a dangerous situation. With that in mind, never leave a dressed and burning candle unattended—that means be *in the room* with your candle spell. If you must leave your candle, extinguish it while saying: "As I extinguish your flame in this realm, I light it in the astral to continue the magic."

There are standard candle-dressing techniques and unique dressing opportunities with each type of candle. Once you pick the type of candle you are going to use in your spell, supercharge it with a custom dressing.

When you dress your candle, you are either pulling something toward you or sending something away, and the initial dressing will reflect that. After this first dressing you can get fancier with carving words and sigils, adding pictures, setting up herbs, and placing crystals. The most successful candle magic experts get really creative when they are dressing candles and setting their lights. Let your imagination be your guide and let's play!

A tip from your Aunt Jacki: A word about glitter and candle dressing—go for it! According to Susan Diamond, proprietor of the Serpent's Kiss magic shop in Santa Cruz, California: "Glitter is like thousands of tiny mirrors, expanding your magic, empowering it and making it bigger than you thought you could." When you add your glitter, the size of the particles matters. If they are too small, they will choke the wick and cause it to gutter out. If they are too big, they can catch fire. Test your glitter, and use a light hand to start until you understand the perfect amount of fab to add to your spell.

THE BIG BOOK OF CANDLE MAGIC

Blessed Candles

Coventry's candles come predressed and blessed as do other candle lines. At Coventry, we do the work for you so that you can jump right into your spell, and we recommend that you tune in to the blessing in the candle to see if it is what you need. Using your pendulum or other divination tool is a quick way to check; an even better way is to psychically tap into the energy and find out if it blends with your intent and empowers it. Dressing a blessed candle fine-tunes a spell's energy and makes it the powerhouse your intent needs to blossom. Use the anointing methods for a pillar candle or get creative and have a little fun with it.

Pillars, Tapers, Chimes, and Votives

Candles not in a container fall into this group of pillars, tapers, chimes, and votives and include a drop-in seven-day candle. (Figure candles have additional dressing options that I will talk about later.) Dressing practices will add a lot to your spell, turning the simple act of setting your intention into a ritual. When you are dressing the candle, let your energy flow with your hands, aligning with your intention and filling it up with your magic.

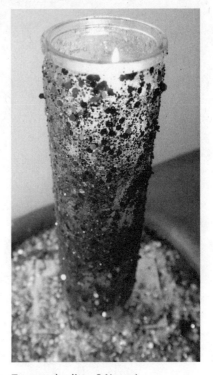

Too much glitter? Never!

You will get your hands dirty when you're dressing candles. Don't be afraid to rub the oil and herbs all over your hands and anoint the candle with flair and emotion. Skip any tools for anointing, and instead use your whole hand for better coverage or your finger for more precise work. Using your own hand is a way to immerse your energy into the spell and the magic into your life. Magic is not a pristine, orderly experience, so throw yourself into the mess of it and have fun!

To Bring Something to You

1. **Toward the center:** Start at either end of the candle and draw the oils and herbs to the center. This represents resources coming to you from every direction.

2. **From heaven to earth:** Start at the top of the candle and anoint it to the bottom. This represents divine support for your spell. It also represents your desire coming closer to you with every moment.

3. **Spiraling it into being:** Spiral your herbs and oils clockwise on the candle from top to bottom. This represents an unraveling of the issue and opening the road for your spell to manifest.

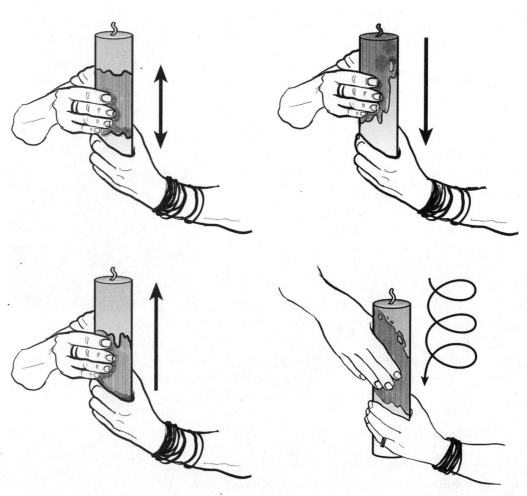

Your intention for how the energy will move in your life is the most important ingredient in anointing your candle.

THE BIG BOOK OF CANDLE MAGIC

4. **Harvesting what you have grown:** With the intention of a successful conclusion of what you have been working on, anoint the candle from the bottom up. This represents the seed you had already planted growing into your life so you are able to harvest the rewards.

To Send Something Away

1. **Clearing it out from the center:** Start at the center of the candle and move your hands outward to either end. This represents clearing from the center out to get to the core of the issue.

2. **Up and out:** Start at the bottom and anoint your candle from the bottom up to the top. This represents removing the energy or issue your spell is for.

3. **Spiraling away the problem:** Start at the bottom and spiral counterclockwise to the top of the candle. This represents unraveling what is keeping the issue entangled in your life.

4. **Burn it away:** With the intent of getting spiritual support to energetically clear the issue, anoint the candle from the top down. This represents a big issue that has enveloped your life, and you are asking for divine support on clearing the energy—burning it all away.

To Bring Balance or Keep Things Steady

Anoint your candle from the ends in and then flip the candle and anoint again from the center out, ending with your hand on the top and bottom. Visualize energy from the earth flowing up your body to your head and back to your hands. Pour that energy into the candle from either end and back into your hands, sending it back to the earth and creating stability.

Figure Candles

Keeping it simple, dress the figure candle the same way you would dress a pillar candle. Getting fancy, you can use your creativity to really have fun with the figure. With all the figure candles out there, the options are endless, and that is a problem. It's difficult to figure out what to do when there are no boundaries. Use the standard candle-dressing techniques as your starting point, and then get inspired with the unique dressing you can do with the standard figure candles.

Seven-knob candles: Dress each knob with a prayer as the next step in manifesting your spell. You can also place a pin in each knob to signal one step closer to your goal.

Cat: Pay special attention to the feet if you are asking the cat energy to hunt something for you. Inscribe your wish on and anoint the cat's tail to make your wish come true.

Cross: Anoint the cross as if you are anointing yourself in the sign of the cross: top, bottom, right, left, and then the center (or head of Jesus). If you are using it as a crossroads, anoint the tip of each arm in a clockwise or counterclockwise motion and the center.

Devil: Dress it like you would a pillar candle.

Human figure/genitalia/lovers/marriage: Anoint the area of the body that your spell will most affect. If you do not have to be specific, use the pillar-anointing method.

Skull: Start your anointing at the base of the skull for influence or creating a mindset. Anoint the eyes for connection, control, or spirit communication. Anoint the top of the crown for healing, and then continue on to anoint the entire skull.

Pyramid: The pillar-anointing rules apply here. Anoint each side of the pyramid, as they can have the same purpose, or you can identify the four pillars of what you are manifesting.

Novena or Seven-Day Candles

I have a deep love for the large devotional candles because you can do so much with them, yet dressing them with herbs and oils is the hardest part.

If you have a pullout candle where the candle comes out of the glass, you can use the dressing techniques from the pillar sections. If you have a standard seven-day candle, there are two schools of thought on dressing them:

1. Put the herbs and oils on top. You can premix the oils and herbs, then apply the mixture or add the ingredients one at a time. You don't need much when you are anointing the top as too many herbs will make a

bonfire out of your candle. Although that may sound cool, it can cause the glass of the seven-day candle to crack and even explode, and that will negatively affect your spell and your flooring.

2. Create a hole one to two inches deep and place the herbs and oils inside. Using a long screwdriver or pick, you will be creating a small hole the width of a screwdriver that is about halfway between the wick and glass. Once the hole is between one and two inches deep, carefully pack the hole with the oils and herbs that align with your candle spell. Again, use a small amount of herbs to prevent a flame flare-up or the clogging of the wick, which will make it gutter out.

Tip from your Aunt Jacki: While dressing my candles, I play chants or carefully chosen music to power up my mood and magic.

This is a slow process and an important part of the ritual. If you try to go too fast, you run the risk of breaking the glass or stabbing yourself with the tool (true story).

The glass container for your seven-day candles allows even more creativity with paint, pictures, and other fun items. Later in this chapter I will go into further detail about sigils and pictures on your candle. When you are dressing the outside glass of the seven-day, glue, glitter, acrylic paint, and permanent markers are your friends. You are limited only by your creativity! I have glued dried flowers onto the glass. I have wrapped the glass in a specific color of

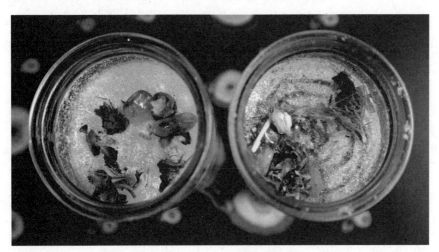

Stones, herbs, and glitter for a seven-day glamour spell.

yarn and woven it in a pattern that supported my spell. You can tie on a blessed knotted cord and even tie two candles together for a love spell. In a fit of joy I covered one glass with glitter and then sealed it with clear acrylic. What can you see yourself dressing your seven-day glass with?

Container Candles

There is a lovely new selection of container candles on the market with fragrances you can't resist. Dress them similar to a seven-day candle and make them magical. If Mahogany Teakwood from Bath & Body Works is a scent you adore, look up the magical uses of those ingredients and make that candle work for you while it smells good. Add more anointing oils and a bit of herbs and you have a dressed designer candle.

While you are being crafty, dress the glass too! All the creativity you would put into a seven-day, pour into your container candle.

Tealights

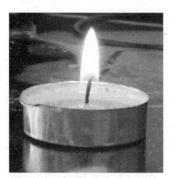

Glitter and oils in one tealight—or several—make for a quick spell.

Let's share a little love for these babies that you can find everywhere from the dollar store to the boutique. So many of the cute candleholders out there are made for tealights, so why not make them magical as they burn for ambience?

Dress your tealight by popping it out of its case, rubbing the herbs and oils on it, then popping it back in. Another of my faves is to pop the candle out of the container and put a few drops of oil in the bottom. The tealight gets molten very quickly, mixing the oils in with the wax nicely. You will get a three-hour spell out of one tealight.

Be careful of the quantity of herbs you put in the tealight, as they can clog the wick, forcing it to go out or, worse, creating a tiny little bonfire that can quickly get out of hand.

SIGILS AND CANDLE SCRIBING

Scribing

Candle scribing is generally used on pillars, tapers, and votives. Container candles lend themselves to using images (see sigil instructions below). If you do nothing else, scribe your intent on your spell candle before you add the oils and herbs. This part of your spell is a commitment from you and firmly sets your intent.

You can scribe a name on the candle to dedicate it to a person, a timeline for when you want it to manifest, a symbol for empowerment, a dollar amount, a personal sigil, or any magical addition you can think of. Scribe the top of the candle for immediate action and the bottom of the candle to keep it secret or for the intent to grow roots in your life. Scribe in a spiral to have it gradually enter your life or find its way to you. Choose the direction of your spiral, up or down, as you would anoint the candle for bringing something in or sending something away.

Use an old ballpoint or gel pen for the familiar control of writing. If you use a new pen, it will immediately become an old pen once the wax clogs it up. Fancy witches I know employ a lovely hatpin dedicated to scribing on candles. You can use your athame or—another of my favorites—a letter

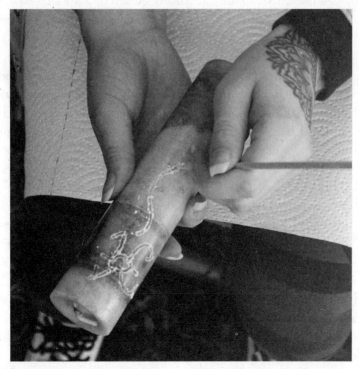

Secure the candle while scribing—with your knees is best—or you can live dangerously like this.

opener. You don't want something too sharp; a dull point will dent the wax, rather than cutting it, and allow your hand to move easier.

Scribing a candle is a very awkward thing. When you set up to scribe your candle, wedge it between two stable items so it won't roll on you. I have locked my knees around the candle, put it on a bunched towel, or when I want to live dangerously, held the candle in my hand until I eventually dropped it and needed to smooth out the dent I just created.

When you are scribing your candle, you can fix mistakes and redo your art by smoothing it over. If you need to keep your spell confidential, you can scribe it, anoint it, and then smooth it out with the intent that the words are moving under the surface. Making a scribe mark disappear can be handled with a little body heat and rubbing the candle until smooth. A more intense redo may require a hair dryer on low.

Sigils

Will my sigil masters stand up! I am totally spoiled by author Laura Tempest Zakroff's sigil skills, such as those found in her book *Sigil Witchery* (Llewellyn, 2018). If you want to dive into sigils, this is worth the read. Laura's technique incorporates intuition, history, art, and a whole bunch of energy to craft unique sigils. She writes, "A sigil is a carved, drawn or painted symbol that is believed to have magical properties. Magick is the art of focusing one's will or intent in order to bring about change. So sigil magic is creating specific symbols to influence one's person, situation, or environment."

Jacki Smith is the candle magic witch.

Sigils are very personal. You are the only one who knows what yours means and what elements are in it to power it up. I will combine symbols to create a blended energy that will aid my magic. For instance, I will take a $, a crown, and a blend of numbers when I am doing a money spell. I also doodle sigils hidden within flowers and shapes to keep my focus on meetings or to bring a certain energy to the meeting.

My personal logo is a sigil with my cat eyeglasses and a flame. When I use that sigil, I am putting my stamp on the magic. Speaking of logos, many corporate logos are sigils. Starbucks is a great example of a sigil as a logo. The founders of Starbucks talk about the siren being a representation of power and protection for their coffee making it across the sea into the port of Seattle.

Amazon's logo is also a sigil to make you smile; FedEx has a sigil with an arrow within the word to represent speedy delivery.

Adding a sigil for a specific outcome is another layer of power in your candle spell. Not only can you scribe it onto the candle; you can also write it out on an anointed paper and carry it with you. I like to call these walking spells; your magic is not stationary and static, it is dynamic. Even when you extinguish your candle for safety's sake, your sigil keeps the magic moving with you all day.

There are a few ways to approach creating a sigil.

1. Personal sigils are an artful combination of the consonants in your name and/or your intent. You would arrange the letters in creative ways to make shapes and patterns.

2. A blend of rune symbols can be layered upon each other create a magical bindrune with a specific purpose. Did you know that the Bluetooth

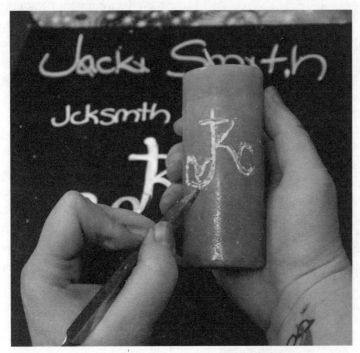

A personal sigil scribed onto your candle powers it up for you alone.

symbol is a bindrune for communication? It uses the initials of the king Harald Bluetooth who united Denmark and Norway in AD 958.

3. A blend of magical symbols can be combined, layered, and arranged to create a sigil to trigger a magical intent. Zakroff teaches a way to create your own list of "word to symbol associations" and use that library to craft your sigils. I love this idea as I don't always connect with the ancient meanings nor can I easily draw them.

4. Astrological symbols can be blended for a love spell. You can also combine the symbols to represent the energy you are manifesting. If you need a little more gumption to speak your mind, for instance, combine Aries and Capricorn. If you want to expand your business, put the symbol of Jupiter and the sun on your candle.

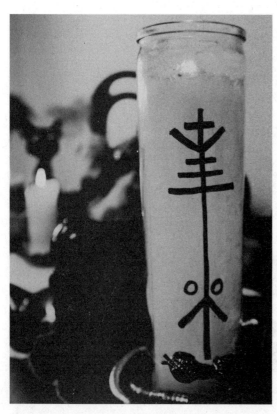

Sharpies, the magical glass-scribing tool.

Draw out your sigil a few times for practice before you scribe it into your candle. You can even draw it with a Sharpie before the carving begins. Sharpies are one of my top ten favorite magical tools, since you can draw on a candle and wipe it off until you get it just right. Then it disappears as you scribe your candle.

What about container candles? Can you scribe or put a sigil on that candle? Yup, use a Sharpie. Whatever you would carve into that wax candle, draw on the glass instead. You get to be a little creative by adding colors, pictures, and/or decoupage to your shabby chic heart's desire. The really cool thing about permanent markers on glass: a little alcohol on a rag takes them right off! Try using the silver or gold markers that add more sparkle to your spell. If you want to be a bit more secretive, use a glue stick that will dry clear, although every time I put a little glue on it I just want to roll it in glitter and make a million mirrors to expand my spell instead.

THE BIG BOOK OF CANDLE MAGIC

IMAGES AND PICTURES

A picture kind of gets right to the point! If you want to influence a specific person—use their picture. That car you have been wanting—boom—show it off to the universe. The place where you want to work? Done—you are hired! That picture tells a tale that a thousand words could not capture because the image that you connect to holds secrets only you and the universe understand. Adding imagery to your spell will laser focus your intent, and when you write out a few directions on the back of that picture, all that energy will fine-tune it and ensure it is moving in the right direction.

Applying images to your candle is a creative process. I always think about what I want to do, what candle I am using, and how that picture fits into my plan. For instance, for a money spell, I printed an image of a $100 bill several times. I then glued the copies to the candleholder to represent unending wealth. When you want to break all contact with someone and get them out of your life, take a picture of them, tear it and burn the edges, and place it under a pair of scissors behind the candle you are burning. You want to get hired fast? Print a copy of your résumé and place the candle you are working on top of it. Is there someone you want to contact or get noticed by? Place your pictures facing each other and secure them to your seven-day candle.

The type of candle you are using will change the way you work with your image. On seven-day glass and container candles, you can glue or secure the image to the glass in some way. You can draw on the glass, creating a vision board right on the container, and add glitter to make something unique.

If you are choosing a pillar candle or taper, your image placement will get even more creative. You can use a candleholder and place the image on or under your holder. Whatever your choice, please

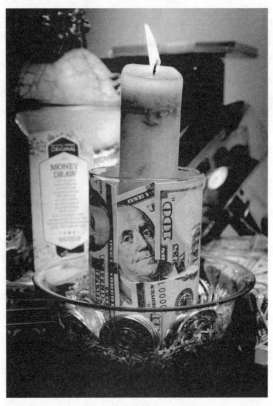

This $100 bill spell was wildly successful.

remember that a candle spell involves fire and pictures are flammable. As safe as you are, that element of fire likes to transform what is around it—i.e., it wants to burn!

Relax and allow your creative juices to flow. Tap into your "Why Is That?" script and use the keywords to influence your image choices to create a picture of your own that represents what you are manifesting. A small vision board is a legit powerful tool. As you layer the images together, you are telling yourself the tale of success with your creativity, your eyes, and your hands. This is also a great place to put your personal sigil for the magic you are creating. Get in touch with your inner magical child and grab a coloring page that represents what you want. The ritual of coloring sends the message of your candle spell's success deep into your soul's core. Place your image on or under your candleholders.

Another method of using images and pictures is to place them on a large surface like a storyboard and position your candle strategically. Grab some large newsprint and draw circles and arrows around the candle and pictures to tell the energy what to do. It's honestly fun and rewarding to move your candle around on the paper to represent your candle spell manifesting. In *Coventry Magic* I share a moving spell where you move a candle closer to draw someone to you. What if you create a road that opens up to your goal and you move your candle along that road, removing or erasing roadblocks along the way?

Craft project from your Aunt Jacki: Look for temporary tattoo or water slide decal paper to print your image or symbol on. You can place that right on a pillar candle as the material will melt away as it burns. You can also use a small amount of acrylic paint directly on a candle and it will melt away before it burns. Too much paint and the wax won't burn away or drip, causing the wick to eventually drown.

A few years ago, a group of moms were concerned about the funding cuts at their school and the division it was creating. We all got together and, using a large piece of easel paper and colored Sharpies, we took turns drawing how we wanted to see the energy flow. There was money flying in from new sources, there were new eyes to see new perspectives, there were kids playing and growing. A path was drawn to show a solution and a heart around the whole mess. It took about eighteen months to manifest, but in the end, this was a successful spell.

You can place your pictures in front of your candle to remind you of what you are going for, reestablishing your spiritual and emotional connection every time you look at it. You can also place the image facing the candle.

Use a seven-day saint candle and place the image in front of it on your altar to show exactly what you need help with.

As I am writing this chapter, I am getting out my craft supplies. I want to decoupage a few seven-day candles for a spell or two. I just discovered that confetti comes in interesting shapes, and that is getting glued onto my candleholder. If the big decorating is not your joy, keep it simple and do the spell—it will be the perfect one for you.

ACCESSORIZING
YOUR SPELL

The candle is my favorite part of the spell. The accessories make the spell a magic party. Just like the shoes can make the outfit, your accessories can make your candle spell even more potent and connected to your intent. The goal is to align as much as possible to the ideal you are creating.

When you add accessories and curios to your spell, you are connecting with your divine child who loves to play and believes in magic. Symbology activates your divine inner child, and at the same time, it brings the literal mind into alignment with the creative mind. The universe does not understand subtlety; it takes everything literally. When you add accessories to your spell, you are embracing the literal and clarifying your spell, not confusing it.

Review the additions you can bring to your spell and get inspired. Pick and choose what calls to you and check in with your pendulum to see if this enhances or takes away from your spell.

DOES ANYONE EVEN KNOW
WHAT TIME IT IS?

The timing of your spell is not a deal breaker, but it can enhance the power of it. I hold strongly to the philosophy that the most powerful time to cast your spell is *when you need it.* That is the moment when you have the biggest emotional commitment to the success of the spell. If you wait too long, doubt creeps in, second-guessing happens, and you tend to think too hard and complicate things. Seize the moment, and if the clock, moon, or astrology is not ideal for your spell, adjust the spell to leverage the energy that is in play. If we are in a waning moon and you need cash, clear the path to getting more cash. If we are in a waxing moon and you want to get someone out of your life, send them to something else they are interested in.

Magic is often about perspective, and the timing of your candle spell is a perfect example of how a new perspective can power up your magic.

Astrologers use a horary chart for divination that shows the astrological alignment "of the hour" or *the moment you ask your question*. Storm Cestavani, my favorite astrologer and podcast cohost, has explained to me that there is a reason you asked at that exact moment and not the day before or later in the evening. It is the astro influences in the moment that tell the tale. This validated my philosophy of filling your magical need in the instant you are inspired to.

If you are more of a planner, there are daily, lunar, and astrological influences that will help you get to your goal if you take a new perspective and leverage the energy of the moment.

Time of Day

> Don't watch the clock; do what it does. Keep going.
>
> —*Sam Levenson*

Starr Casas, author of *Old Style Conjure: Hoodoo, Rootwork, & Folk Magic* (Weiser Books, 2017), taught me about working magic around the clock. Mama Starr doesn't ascribe to watching the phases of the moon; she watches the clock instead. When the hands are going down, she does clearing magic, when the hands are going up, she does increase or attraction magic. That's it. It's straightforward and clear. From noon to 5:59 the hands of the clock say clearing magic is better, from 6 to 11:59 the clock will support magic that creates increase. You have two cycles in the day to do that magic: a.m. and p.m.

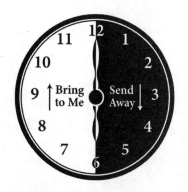

Don't have time to wait for the moon? Use the clock.

Days of the Week

Each day in the week lends a bit of magical assistance. What's happening on the day of your spell? How will the energetic vibration of that day affect your candle magic?

Sunday is from the Latin *Solis dies*, which means "sun's day." Sunday is a good day for healing and prosperity magic as it enhances magic concerning authority, strength, divine power, and learning. Friendship spells are good on Sunday.

Monday is from the Latin *Lunae dies*, which means "moon's day." This is a good day for love spells that affect the family. Clearing and healing spells that work with emotions, dreams, intuition, and spiritual growth are also good on a Monday.

Tuesday is from the Latin *Martis dies*, which means "Mars's day." This is a good day for protection spells that need courage, strength, or war and conflict resolution. Healing spells that need vitality and strength to carry on are supported by Tuesday energy.

Wednesday is from the Latin *Mercurii dies*, which means "Mercury's day." This is a good day for clearing and healing spells for self-improvement, divination, mystical insight, and resourcefulness.

Thursday is from the Latin *Jovis dies*, which means "Jupiter's day." This is a good day for prosperity spells for money, success, and luck. It is also good for protection spells for legal matters, loyalty, and endurance.

Friday is from the Latin *Veneris dies*, which means "Venus's day." This is a good day for all love spells, including for fertility, partnership, and friendship. Love spells can also include your love of art, music, and anything that brings your soul pleasure.

Saturday is from the Latin *Saturni dies*, which means "Saturn's day." This is a good day for prosperity and healing spells that need a boost of motivation, understanding, and will. This is also an excellent day for clearing and banishing spells.

When the Moon Is Right

The moon is never wrong, so this is all about using the pull of the moon to power up your spell. There are officially eight phases of the moon; new, waxing crescent, first quarter, waxing gibbous, full moon, waning gibbous, last quarter, waning crescent. This twenty-eight-day cycle, if you tie your magical working to it 100 percent, can limit the time span you can do any spell. Think about the spell you want to do, and then look up where the moon phase is right now. You just need to tailor your spell to that phase to get the result you want.

Moon Phase	Keywords	For Increase	For Decrease
New	Planting, new beginning, new thoughts, revealing, new possibilities, intention setting, planning, clearing the old and outdated	This is the perfect time to plant the seed of what results you want and set your intention for this cycle through the next new moon.	Set your intention of what your overall goal is, focusing on what you will be gaining from the intent. Focus on what will be coming in, displacing what you want to go away. Cast for protection against any backlash from your spell.
Waxing Crescent	Building upon hopes and dreams, initiative, fresh new energy, budding ideas, planning, detail work, beginnings	Plan your work so you can work your plan. Think about all the steps you will experience while your magic manifests. Fill your spell with fresh energy and new ideas to accomplish your goal.	Grab this energy and fill yourself with it. Allow the waxing crescent to fill you with new ideas and fresh perspective on your issue. Use this energy to come up with a plan of how life will get better as you displace what needs to leave with this fresh energy and new perspective.
First Quarter	Action, building upon what has begun, grounding and rooting, creativity, bravery, momentum, overcoming challenges	Charge this spell up! This is a prime time to grab this momentum and ricochet into success. Ground yourself in what you are manifesting and take action toward your goal.	Use the momentum of the first quarter to get grounded in everything you are grateful for, the blessings in your life, and vibrate to that. What needs to be cleared cannot exist in the state of connection to your blessings.

Moon Phase	Keywords	For Increase	For Decrease
Waxing Gibbous	Do the work, evaluate, refine, nurture, wait, patience, building pressure, aligning with the universe	Start acting as if what you want has already manifested and nurture its arrival. Breathe and know that you are in the final stages of bringing to you what you want. Don't let go!	You are at the tail end of your struggle. Define in detail what your life will be like without the energy you are clearing and shift your energy to that ideal. What no longer serves you will start falling away.
Full Moon	Pinnacle of energy, blessings, joy, healing, completion, empowered, psychic, celebration, fruitful	Grab all the energy and pull it into your spell, charging up your intent to a place where you can feel your success. This is the last moment to do an increased spell for the next two weeks. Tune in to your future and see what this blessing will look like as it manifests.	Grab all the energy of the full moon and use it to push out what you need to clear and fill yourself up with empowerment, joy, gratitude, blessings, and connection with your higher purpose.
Waning Gibbous	Harvest, receive, release, nurture, turn inward, stillness, sharing, teaching, counting abundance	Focus on what you have already accomplished in this area and harvest it; it is more than you think it is. Pay forward what you are working to manifest through service to others and sharing blessings.	Release, release, release. Turn your clearing spell into a stepped release to ensure you are complete in your clearing. As you release, define what you are receiving in place of what you are giving up.

continued

Moon Phase	Keywords	For Increase	For Decrease
Last Quarter	Let go, readjust, clear, reflect, change, past, new perspective, breakdown, decompose	List what has not worked in your life that brought you to manifesting this new idea. Allow your perception on this to evolve and adjust to a new understanding, and release the limiting energy in your life. Forgive yourself and others for what limits you are finding.	Break apart what you are clearing into smaller steps that you are letting go of. Understand that what you are clearing has served you in the past and, as you clear it, you are left with a blessing of some type.
Waning Crescent	Restore, reflection, rest, surrender, empty, conclusion, release, let go	Let go of the outcome of your plan. Surrender your wants to the divine and let them cocreate with you. Cast for a clearing of old thought patterns that stop you from intuitively knowing what your next step is.	This is time for a total release and clearing on every level. You are ready to let go and let the big lesson become wisdom. Reflect on what you have learned in this process.

Cheat Sheet on the Phase of the Moon

I lose track of what phase the moon is in all the time. I can look at my calendar and then go outside, look at the moon, and wonder what phase it is. So I created a cheat sheet that I keep in my wallet to ensure I continue to impress and look witchy at every moment.

The new moon rises and sets with the sun, thus we cannot see it.
 When you see the crescent of the moon on the right side, it is waxing, heading toward the full-moon phase.

The full moon rises as the sun sets and sets as the sun rises.
 When you see the crescent of the moon on the left side, it is waning, heading toward the new-moon phase.

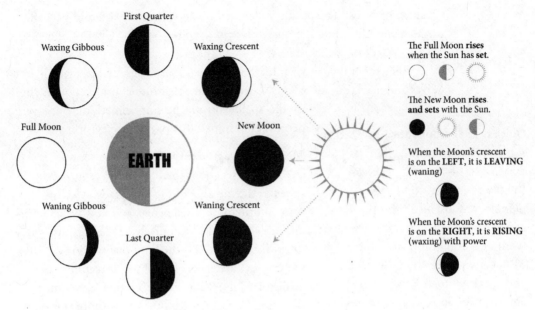

First Quarter

Waxing Gibbous

Waxing Crescent

The Full Moon **rises** when the Sun has **set**.

Full Moon

New Moon

EARTH

The New Moon **rises and sets** with the Sun.

Waning Gibbous

Waning Crescent

When the Moon's crescent is on the **LEFT**, it is **LEAVING** (waning)

Last Quarter

When the Moon's crescent is on the **RIGHT**, it is **RISING** (waxing) with power

Lunar cheat sheet.

Astrological Influences

Moon energy rules our emotions and emotional responses to the world. It is seen as a symbol of magic, and maybe that is because our emotions are a big part of our magic. The phase and the astrological sign it is in will influence the vibration of the energy around us, making it worthwhile to check your ephemeris and see if your spell needs a bit of adjusting to fully employ the energy that is already abundant. In the astrological index, you will find the magic that is activated as the moon travels through the signs. The moon travels through all twelve of the signs of the zodiac in twenty-eight days. It is in each sign for 2–2.5 days, giving you time to get your candle spell supplies in order as you wait for the perfect moment.

Retrogrades

Retrogrades, especially Mercury, get everyone into a tailspin, and we get to blame all tomfoolery on that aspect. The important thing to remember about a retrograde is the prefix—*re-*. Sure, if you are feeling shaky, postpone your spell if there is a retrograde, but you may be waiting weeks, months, or even years. The retrogrades to be concerned with are the inner planets: Mercury,

Venus, or Mars. The planets whose orbits lie within the asteroid belt affect your daily life, while the outer planets—Jupiter, Saturn, Uranus, and Neptune—affect the wider society.

Remember that retrogrades show us what is not working optimally in our lives and needs our attention. When you take that into consideration in your candle spell, you are healing something on a very deep level to hopefully not have to revisit it again.

Mercury retrograde: Occurs three to four times a year and lasts about three weeks. *Review, review, review* is the message of the retrograde. Mercury rules information, intelligence, and how we communicate to the world and ourselves. Mercury also rules short-distance travel—the kind that we do every day to manage the details of our lives. Perceptions can be distorted during Mercury retrograde. We may interpret things incorrectly, speak without clarity, and jump to conclusions. Review, renew, revise during Mercury retrograde before you build your candle spell.

Venus retrograde: Occurs about every eighteen months and will last approximately six weeks. Venus rules love and beauty, how we give and receive love, and where we find comfort and support within ourselves and others. Venus retrograde brings mixed messages, confusing and wildly shifting emotions, and may make your love life feel stagnant. Love, family, breakup, and new-money spells are negatively influenced by Venus retrograde. Reflect, relate, remain, renew during Venus retrograde before you build your candle spell.

Mars retrograde: Occurs about every twenty-six months and will last approximately ten weeks. Mars rules our will and courage and activates our fiery and passionate side. Mars governs how we assert ourselves, which can be aggression or bravery and self-empowerment. Mars retrograde brings sluggish, unmotivated energy and makes us struggle for action in a tangible way. Rest, reflect, return during Mars retrograde before you build your candle spell.

Eclipse

There are between four and eight eclipses per year; a solar eclipse occurs on a new moon and a lunar eclipse occurs on a full moon. During an eclipse, avoid candle spells that attract, increase, or manipulate energy to your advantage. I really don't recommend any magic during this time, but if you do your astrological homework, candle spells for uncrossing, spiritual cleansing, or to remove energy can all be done during an eclipse.

If you are an expert astrologer, you may decide to look at all aspects that are occurring during an eclipse and weigh how they interact with your natal chart to build your candle spell from that information. But if you are an astrological layperson like me, leave that energy alone. Don't fiddle with something you don't fully grasp.

THIS IS DEDICATED TO THE ONE I LOVE— NAME PAPERS

Name papers are a classic conjure technique to connect to the energy of a specific person and direct your spell to them. This doesn't work on perfect strangers; you need to have some kind of connection with them within two degrees of separation. If you know who owns the company you want to work for but have never met them or their inner circle, a name paper is not going to give you the link you are looking for.

If the person you are bringing into your spell is very close to you, saying their name can be enough to make that connection. A picture or copy of a picture makes an excellent name paper especially when you write their name on it. A business card handed directly to you can be used as a name paper. A tissue or something that touched their body (*ewww*) can be used in place of a name paper. If you don't have any of these, make a name paper.

To create a name paper, tear a piece of paper on all four sides. Write down their full name and add any other defining information about them: birth date, astrological sign, phone number, address, screen name, URL, etc. Hold the paper in the palm of your hand and knock on that paper three times to wake up the connection to that person. Whisper their name into the paper and remind them of the connection you have to them. (*Johnny Jones, I worked with you last year, and we shared a workstation.*) Hold the paper in both hands and visualize this person, their face, voice, and energy. Push that energy into the paper. You now have a name paper that can be added to your spell.

I assume, at this point, you will use the name paper only for beneficial purposes.

CRYSTALS AND STONES

Stones are beautiful, they are high vibration, they are magic, and now you have a reason to buy more—to use them in your candle spells! When I got my first baby stones, I would make patterns with them. Intuitively, I would arrange them in a pleasing shape then look up their meaning. That was how I got to know my babies and they got to know me: we learned how our energy worked together.

When including your stones in your spell, sit with them before you place them. (If this is a brand-new stone, cleanse it of any other person's energy or the trauma of being pulled out of the earth.) Telepathically ask your stones if they are willing to be a part of the magic you are crafting. The spirit or primal energy in a stone is very potent; it has been on this earth since the beginning, has seen a lot of things, and has some definite opinions on how it will bring its magic to you. Getting agreement from your stone makes your spell that much more powerful, but not getting agreement can make some of your magic fizzle out.

Grab your "Why Is That?" page and ask your stone what part of this transformation it is willing to be a part of. For fun, intuitively pick a few stones and ask for their participation before you look up how they can be used in your spell. You will be magically surprised! If your stone does not feel like it is in alignment with an existing definition, go with what your stone is telling you. It is the master of its own energy.

Magical experiment from your Aunt Jacki: If you can't believe that stones have the type of energy you can commune with, do this experiment. Go walking in nature and ask to be guided to a rock that wants to help you with your magic. Then try not to find it. Last time I did this, I kicked the stone and almost tripped. Today, when I am out in the wilds, or the almost wilds you get in the city, there are rocks that want to be put in my pocket. I leave 99 percent of them for the next rock lover, but it is a joy to commune with them.

How to Use Stones in Your Candle Spell

Creativity is the name of the game when including stones in your candle spells. There are many stones and shapes to choose from. Natural rough, tumbled, natural point, carved point, obelisk, pyramid, skull, palm stones, animal shapes, angels, hearts, and more—your choice is most often dictated by what you have on hand, but if you are shopping for your spell, think about what purpose it will serve and whether the shape or style helps or hurts your intention.

Any stone you add to your spell has a job and a purpose. It will direct energy, be a supportive vibration, act as a power source, or bring a new vibration.

Energy directors: You can use quartz points to move energy away from or toward your spell. In a spell that represents change or movement in your life, use your energy director stones to signal that movement.

Supportive vibrations: Stones can represent people in the spell, the energetic shift you are intending, or an intensifier of a specific energy to support your spell. If this stone represents a person, choose the stone according to the astrological sign or personality of the person you are targeting. If this stone represents an energy shift, use the stone that represents the final goal. If this stone is an intensifier, you can place it on a picture to send that energy directly while your candle spell manifests.

Power sources: Big spells deserve energy generators to keep them going. Place a large quartz cluster under your altar to keep the energy moving. Place a slab under your candleholder, or surround the candleholder with energizing stones. Crystals and high vibration stones are not the only power sources. Spells that need grounding can be energized by stones that do exactly that.

New vibration: If your candle and dressing choices don't quite match the intent you're crafting a spell for, a crystal can add the finishing touch to bringing your energy into alignment.

See the Crystal and Stone Index in the back of the book to help choose stones for your spell.

Crystal Grids

Grids are another way to incorporate crystal energy into your candle spell. My first crystal and candle grid did not use one of those lovely laser-cut templates you can find now. I placed the stones and the candles around my home while creating an energetic grid to cleanse and protect. The candles started and defined the energy flow; the crystals were charged with that energy and held it in place. This was the reverse of the stone influencing the spell. This time the spell programmed the stone. I have done this with clear quartz, rose quartz, selenite, and fieldstones.

Home Protection Candle and Stone Grid

Need:

Eight white candles— either votives dressed with spiritual cleansing oil or blessed votives

Eight stones dressed with protection oil

1. Starting in the center of your home, set up all candles in their holder and stones. Dress the candles and stones while inviting in your guardian protectors. Pair up the candles and stones. One for the heart of the home, one for each direction, one for above, one for below, and one to connect the energy. State your words of power over your candles and stones.

2. Light one votive to be your heart candle. Place its companion stone with it. Light your connection candle from the heart candle, and touch the connection stone to the heart stone. Place the connection candle and stone in one hand and carry the south votive and stone to the south wall of your home.

3. Place the candle and stone in the south, say your words of power, light the candle with the connection candle, and touch the connection stone to the south stone. Walk clockwise through your home back to the heart candle.

4. Take the west candle and stone, with the connection candle and stone, clockwise past the south wall, to the west wall of your home. Place them in a safe spot, say your words of power, light the west candle with the connection candle, and touch the connection stone to the west stone. Walk clockwise through your home back to the heart candle.

5. Take the north candle and stone, with the connection candle and stone, walk clockwise past the south wall and west wall to the north wall of your home. Place them in a safe spot, say your words of power, light the north candle with the connection candle, and touch the connection stone to the north stone. Walk clockwise through your home back to the heart candle.

6. Take the east candle and stone, with the connection candle and stone, walk clockwise past the south wall, west wall, and north wall to the east wall of your home. Place them in a safe spot, say your words of power, light the east candle with the connection candle, and touch the connection stone to the east stone. Walk clockwise through your home back to the heart candle.

7. Touch the connection stone to the heart stone and the flames of the heart and connector candles together. Say your words of power, light the above candle with the connector candle, and touch the above stone with the connector stone. Light the below candle with the connector candle, and touch the below stone with the connector stone.

8. Touch the connection stone to the heart stone and the flames of the heart and connector candles together. Walk the above and below candles, clockwise, past all of the directional candles. Set them with the heart and connector candles and stones in the center of the house. Say your words of power one more time.

9. Sit in meditation and visualize the grid in and around your home, filling it with divine protection energy and displacing any discordant energy. When you feel the grid is firmly in place, extinguish the candles one by one in the same order you lit them. Place the stones where they will not be disturbed and the candles on your altar.

10. Relight the candles every day until they are consumed to anchor the grid in your home.

I have set up large candle and crystal grid spells for creativity in an entire building by using a variety of stones. I have done communication grids with carved skull stones and selenite. I have created romance grids with garnet, joy and harmony grids for family functions with amethyst, and prosperity grids for my office with large quartz and citrine. I would recharge them regularly, and they last until I pull up the stones and clear them.

Sacred geometry grids, like the flower of life, can give you a head start in manifesting your spell. Simply adding your candle to the center of the grid with crystals strategically placed around it draws the energy of sacred geometry into your spell. The addition of grid magic is a serious energy boost and feels like magical play to me. Letting your creative magic juices flow with grids is a big part of their power.

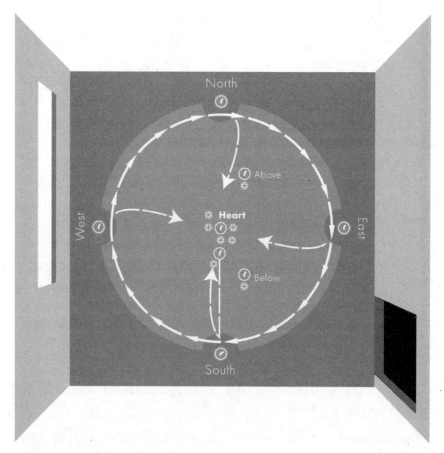

Candle and crystal grid for clearing and protection.

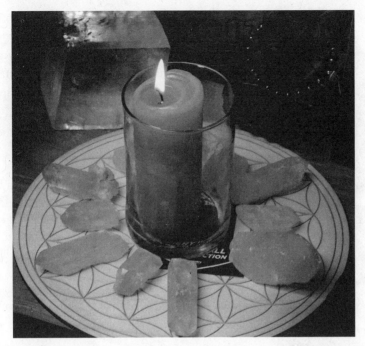

The flower of life grid amps up any spell. All you need is your imagination. As a protection spell it will keep all interfering energies away.

Pendulum Magic

Pendulums are the easiest tool to confirm agreement with stones, especially if the one you work with is made of stone. There are other styles of pendulums—metal, glass, orgonite, to name a few—but I find that the stone pendulums work best for me. Maybe that's because I use them for magic as well as divination. I have included more information on how to divine for your candle magic in the section on pendulums in the first part of this book.

Pendulums can be a way to move energy as well as divine it. If you have a spell that needs a boost, choose a stone pendulum that complements the spell and gently spin it over the candle clockwise to pull more energy into it. If you have a spell to clear something, gently spin the pendulum counterclockwise. Gently start the spin and let the momentum of the energy in the spell speed it up or slow it down. If it slows too fast, manually speed up the spin to move the energy.

If a candle gutters out for a nontechnical reason, use the pendulum with a counterclockwise spin to clear the energy of the candles. Sometimes that is enough to reset your spell and relight the candle. If not, clear your personal energy and do a reading to see if you need to start over with a different candle spell before you finish this one. If you are restarting the same candle spell, you may need to manipulate the candlewick and wax to help it get going.

TAROT

Are you telling a fortune, casting a spell, or both? Tarot and candle spells go together like peanut butter and chocolate. Each is wonderful on its own, but together, they are a treat.

There are two paths to add tarot to your candle magic.

1. Use the messages of the cards to add to your candle spell.

2. Use your candle spell to enhance or counter the results of your tarot reading.

Adding Tarot to Your Candle Spell

Laying out a tarot spread tells your psyche, the universe, your divine allies, and your spirit exactly the outcome you are looking for. Three cards spread out in front of your candles are all you need to start adding tarot to your candle magic.

First card: where you are now

Second card: the process, or what you need to break through

Third card: the conclusion of your spell

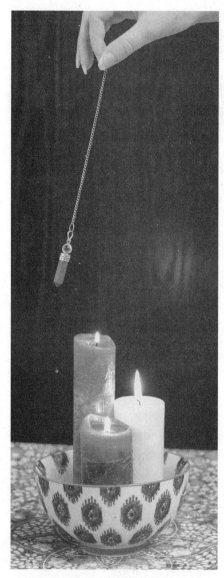

Use a pendulum to check the energy of your spell before, during, and after.

Having a deck dedicated to candle spells is a fine idea, since they may get a little waxy. Not worrying about using them later lets you get a little creative. I have tied three cards to a seven-day candle. I have placed the cards under the

THE BIG BOOK OF CANDLE MAGIC

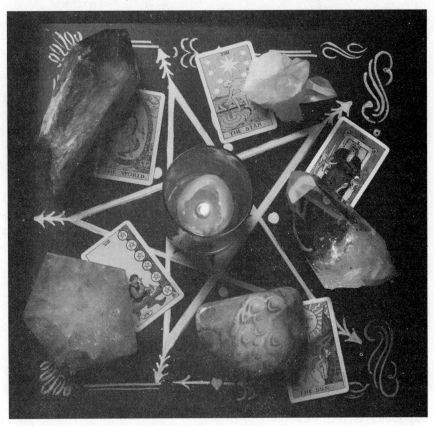

Candles, tarot, crystals, and sigils—this spell is loaded.

plate that held my candles. I have made a photocopy of the cards, written on the paper, and placed it under a candle that will drip.

Try this: Sit with your "Why Is That?" list and a deck of tarot cards. Start to pull out the cards that resonate with your deeper need and final intent for your spell. When they are laid out with your candle and other ingredients, start to play.

Adding a Candle Spell to Your Tarot Reading

I have been thrown off balance by tarot readings and wanted to avoid what the cards foretold. Perhaps you have too. Time for a candle spell! I record what the cards are and set them on my altar to decide what magical action to take with my candle spells. For the parts of the reading I want to counter the effects of, I will do a clearing candle spell. For the parts I want to enhance, I will set up a candle spell specific to the reading. This is one of the few times I will do two spells at the same time, since, really, they are two parts of the same spell.

On the flip side, adding tarot to your candle spell can be a fast way to your goal. Scan through the Tarot Index to choose the tarot cards that can fast track your spell.

CHARMS, CURIOS, AND ORGANIC ITEMS

These items are not herbs, oils, or stones, and yet they are useful in many candle spells. This is not an exhaustive list, as there are things in your kitchen and keepsake box that you will be inspired to use in future candle spells. However, you can use this quick list as a starting point and as inspiration to repurpose other items in your junk drawer.

Black Cat Hair

Prosperity, Protection, Love

Used for luck, cat energy, seduction, hunting energy. It can be made into black cat oil for luck and protection against bad luck. Always gather hair naturally shed by the cat.

Cascarilla

Protection, Clearing

Made from eggshells, this natural chalklike powder can be employed to define a sacred space, to call in divine energies, as a protection against evil entering the space, and in purification rituals.

Crossroads

Prosperity, Protection, Love, Clearing, Healing

Crossroads are a place where two or three roads intersect with no visible dead ends. This is the space of magic where all potential lives and all things are connected. Each direction at a crossroads is a new potential. If you can't get to a crossroads to perform your spell or make an offering, you can create your own with crossed skeleton keys, a cross figure candle, an equal-armed cross of wood, or, in a pinch, a drawing of a cross.

Crown

Prosperity, Healing

Crown motifs symbolize success, recognition for your work, and connection to your divine self.

Dice

Prosperity

Use in spells where you need the odds to be in your favor.

Feathers

Love, Clearing, Healing

Use to sweep away negative energy. Feathers help you rise above the situation and take a bird's-eye view. They can also bring messages and allow you to fly free of a situation. Employ only feathers that are either legally purchased or are legal to own—the rules around this are more complicated than you think.

Flowers

Prosperity, Love, Clearing, Healing

A fresh bunch of flowers brings the energy of abundance and life to your spell. Use to charge or recharge a prosperity spell. The love language of flowers can send a message to your target. Use white flowers to cleanse a space. Bring flowers into healing work as an additional life force. These can also be offerings to spirit and ancestors.

High John the Conqueror Root

Prosperity, Love, Healing

Also known as jalap or Ipomoea jalapa, the root of a kind of morning glory, this root powers up your magic and brings confidence, cunning, and luck. Is used for virility in men and libido in women.

Horseshoe

Prosperity, Protection

Used to attract good luck and protection against evil and ill will, horseshoes hung with prongs up collect luck and keep it in place. Some superstitions say that a horseshoe with prongs down passes luck to everyone who passes under it.

Lodestone

Prosperity, Love

A natural magnetic stone used in spells where you are attracting anything to you. Use magnetic sand to activate the magic of magnetism. Two lodestones can be used in love spells to bring a lover or strengthen a marriage. Paired lodestones are also used in fidelity spells.

Magnetic Sand

Prosperity

Use with a lodestone or magnet to activate attraction.

Money

Prosperity, Protection

Any money used in a spell will attract the energy of prosperity and commerce. But specific coins have particular energies:

Mercury dime: Use for good fortune, communication, protection against curses and tricks laid against you.

Sacagawea dollar: Use to open the road, especially to a new home.

Susan B. Anthony dollar: Use for any spell that increases the power and independence of a woman. Excellent for women in business.

Silver dollar: Use to attract prosperity.

Two-dollar bill: Use to attract luck in a business venture.

Wooden nickel or token: Use when you need people to believe in you and your vision. Also useful in spells when you need to trick people into believing you.

Fake money: The bigger the bill, the better to represent attracting abundance in your life. Use it as a petition paper to write your intent on to power up the pull of money.

Shredded money: Use in money spells to represent an abundance of money.

Poker or gambling chip: Use in Luck spells.

Railroad Spike

Protection, Clearing

Use in protection, clearing, grounding, and anchoring spells. Place in the four corners of your property to create a protective barrier. Employ in a cleansing to pull the energy off of you and into the ground. Apply in a prosperity spell to anchor abundance into your life. These can also function in a ritual to stay grounded.

Red Flannel

Protection, Clearing, Prosperity, Love, Healing

Used in mojo bags and altar cloths to represent the quickening of magic that occurs when heaven and earth meet.

Salt

Protection, Clearing

Salt can create a barrier between the spiritual and mundane and against negative energies entering a sacred space. It is also used to draw negative energy from your body, mind, and spirit. Particular types of salt can be put to various uses:

Pink Himalayan: Clearing and energizing. Use in salt baths or scrubs to pull out energetic impurities and replace them with a higher energy. Helps in healing issues of self-love.

Sea: This is the preferred salt for cleaning your tools and scrying mirrors. Brings blessings of health.

Black: Primarily use it to create a protective barrier. When placed under the head of your bed, it is excellent in preventing nightmares and pulling any mental influence off of you. Also excellent in stopping gossip.

Scissors

Protection, Clearing

Cleansed scissors can be used to cut hooks and drains. Place open scissors under the head of your bed, pointing toward the head, to protect from anyone entering your dreams and to cut away any mental influence. Open scissors near your front door prevent anyone who intends harm from entering your home.

Shells

Prosperity, Love, Clearing, Healing

Depending on the shell, it can represent money, divinity, messages, fertility, and clearing of your energy. Each shell has its own energy like herbs or stones, making them an active living addition to a spell.

Skeleton Key

Protection, Clearing, Healing

Holding the key to anything gives you the power and authority over your own life. Skeleton keys stand in as the key to wisdom, riches, freedom, and love.

Skull (Human Style)

Love, Healing

Human skulls carved out of crystal or stone, cast in plaster or other materials, or made out of a variety of components represent the wisdom of the ages, ancestors, and communication. Use in spells where you need more information and clear communication between people or with spirit. Can also be used as a representation of a specific spirit guide.

Tobacco

Protection, Clearing, Healing

Tobacco is first and foremost a sacred offering to spirit to honor them and promote well-being. It can be used to connect to divinity and offer your prayers and to cleanse a space or person of attachments. Most magical practitioners use tobacco on its own, separate from a magical blend, making it more of a stand-alone organic charm. If your relationship with tobacco inspires its addition to your blend, then use that wisdom to create a powerful spell.

FLARE FOR DRAMA

When life hands you a bucket full of BS, sometimes you need a flare for drama to counter all that negativity. Expressing that drama in your daily life is not effective or healthy—but saving it for your spell can be.

When crafting a candle spell and ritual around something that is deeply emotional, stressful, and traumatic, give yourself a big bang moment that clears the trauma and the accompanying emotions. Elevating your spell to a ritual allows you to speak to every level of the self and spirit and can move the stuck energy out of your physical body.

Breaking Glass

Breaking glass is a big, shocking, emotional release. You are causing a huge disruption in the vibration around you. It wakes your energy up, giving you notice to pay attention to what you are doing. It helps you shake up that inner issue holding you back or that you are holding on to. If you choose to purposefully break glass, start with caution; use gloves, safety goggles, and other protective gear.

Seven-day candles are the traditional choice for glass-breaking spells, yet the glass container candles that are popular today will work too. There are two standard choices when you break the glass: before you burn the candle and after. Your choice of times will be based on your perspective.

> **Make the break and clear:** Breaking the glass before you burn the candle has the energy of ripping off the Band-Aid and then managing the fallout. Add this cathartic moment to breakup spells, breaking curse spells, removing influence, breaking a bad habit, blockbusting, removing someone from your life, and removing hooks and drains.

> Dress and bless your candle, set up the entire spell, and instead of lighting the candle first, you will put the candle in a paper bag and smash it.

> The wax in the container candle is softer than pillar candle wax; in essence it requires a candleholder to burn without becoming a puddle

fast. If you break the glass first, you will have to carefully pick out the shards and then place the candle in another holder or find an alternate way for the candle to be consumed or disposed of. Throwing it into a bonfire, putting it in a large metal bowl, or even throwing the whole thing away in the garbage and cleansing yourself after it is disposed of are options.

Doing the work and making the break: Doing the spell first, making sure all parts are in place for the break, and then finishing it off with smashing the glass give a lovely cathartic finale. Add this flare of drama to spells where you are finishing an unpleasant task, step-by-step moving someone out of your life, going through a divorce, going through a healing process, doing a long-term cleansing, or breaking a bad habit.

Dress and bless your candle, set up your spell, and start the candle burning. Do the day-to-day work you need to support the spell. When the spell and candle are finished, put the candle in a paper bag and smash it. You can do this in a garbage can or dumpster for easy disposal.

Think about what variation on this you would add to your spell. How would you customize this? Would you smash it partway through? Would you throw it into a dumpster to smash it? Make sure with any method you use to be safe and careful—broken glass can be dangerous.

Cascading Candles

Cascading candles can be like a candle garden of pillars lit together in a single candleholder so they pool their wax together. Cascading candles can also be a series of candles you light one after another; as one candle burns out, you light the next one from the flame of the previous candle.

A candle garden on a large, deep platter or baking sheet with sides gives you an opportunity to read the wax as it drips and pools. Pillar candles placed close together will intensify the heat of the flame, causing the candles to melt faster. Candles of varying colors pool around each other and blend in a magical way. Multiple candles in one spell become a story of your magic and intent, and the melting wax may tell its own story about how it will manifest.

A candle series also tells a story. You can use the same candle in repetition to reenergize your spell for an amount of time. You can use a series of different candles as a progressive spell that represents the transformation you are manifesting. Votives are a popular choice for a candle series. Coventry's Blessing Kits are an example of a cascading spell. You can burn them either together or one by one and achieve the same results.

Flash

Flash paper and Vesta powder are two easy ways to put a little bang into your candle spell. Safer than breaking glass, a bit of flash can create a big shift in energy that fast-forwards your spell. Flash can add energy or break a curse depending on how you define its purpose in your spell.

Flash paper is often used by sleight-of-hand magicians for a big effect and misdirection. It is made from a special tissue treated with nitric acid that can produce a brilliant flame or flash when it comes in contact with a heat source like a lighter, match, or candle.

For candle spells you can add flash paper when you are transforming something like your luck or clearing something like a web of lies. It can also be used to give a boost of energy to your intent by writing your words of power on flash paper and lighting it with your candle flame. Flash paper goes up in a flash, so to be on the safe side, use caution where and when you light it. Stay away from flammable items, and maybe outside is the best place to do this.

Vesta powder is an older magical tool made of potassium nitrate (saltpeter) and cornstarch. Formerly called chasing powder or flash powder, Vesta powder is used to empower or clear. It breaks the energetic hold that negative energies or entities have on you and clears your energy in a flash to help you power up and manifest your intent. Vesta powder is very flammable so must be stored carefully and used in an open area. Do not touch your face, eyes, mouth, or nose when using Vesta powder. Immediately wash with soap and water if you get some of the powder on your skin.

Burning Spells

Many rituals through the ages include adding offerings to the fire as an appeal for blessing, to create a personal transformation, or to purge what is ready to be released. You are already burning a candle, so why not use the transformational energy of flame to burn something as part of your spell? When you use the flame of your candle for spellwork, you are widening the scope of the magic and making a larger spell.

To bring something to you, burn your petition paper at the beginning of the spell with an offering of herbs to send your desire to the divine. You can also burn your petition paper at the end of the spell in thanks and offering.

To release something, write it out, and at the end of your candle spell, burn it as a final release. You can also burn it at the beginning of your candle spell and use the spell to support continuing the release over time.

To empower transformation, burn what you are releasing and use the ashes to bless the next candle or part of the ritual. Once when I was facilitating a public ritual, I brought out my big cauldron, added a selection of blessed candles, and we burned something to release or transform. We then used the ashes in a second part of the ritual to bring something into being.

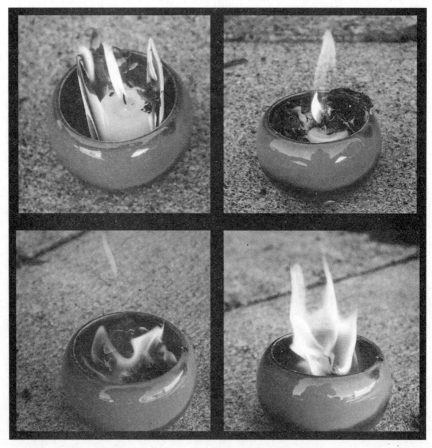

Burning bowl to release your spell. Let it go and let the universe make it happen.

We burned messages of hate, added the ashes to paint, and created paintings filled with love.

Burning bowl ceremonies are another example of a burning spell and make a lovely way to release your past. This ceremony can be done alone or with a trusted group of magical companions. Working as a group intensifies the commitment to the release, thus increasing the intensity of the magic. There are a few simple steps to a burning bowl ceremony, and it all begins with a candle and is best done outside.

1. Choose a candle. Most often this is a votive so it will be consumed by the end of the ceremony. You will need a dressed plain votive or a blessed votive for spiritual cleansing, banishing, or releasing. Put the candle in the center of a metal bowl or a tempered glass bowl large enough for papers to burn next to the candle.

2. Meditate on the candle flame with the intent of releasing what is limiting your growth. Let your mind and emotions drift, allowing what is ready to be released to float to the top.

3. Write what you are releasing on a slip of paper. Visualize what you are letting go of moving from your energy and body into the paper. Say an affirmation of release of your own or use this example:

   Today I release what I don't want from my past. I forgive myself and trust in the forgiveness of divine love. I let go of feelings of self-blame, shame, and guilt. I release any connection or hook from or to another. I allow the sacred rhythm of life to heal and renew me. I open my heart to release what no longer serves my highest good, and I am blessed with love, peace, joy, and harmony.

4. Light your paper from the candle flame and drop into the bowl. Watch the smoke rise and pull with it any resistance you had to letting go. Watch as the smoke dissipates as you become free of the burden you released.

5. Restate the affirmation and focus on gratitude by making a list of what you are grateful for and how that gratitude will support your transformation after this release.

6. When you feel complete, extinguish the candle and dispose of the remains in a garbage depository away from your home or work.

Combining your candle spell with a burn creates an empowerment or finality to your intent. It is an easy supplement to your candle spell and can be added at any time.

Putting Out the Flame

To blow or to snuff—that is the question. You can make the act of extinguishing your candle a part of the spell, and you can even make it a bit dramatic. My normal candle spell etiquette is to lovingly blow the candle out. I am not in the camp that says never to blow out the candle as you will be canceling the spell. My magic—and yours as well—is much stronger stuff and cannot be dispersed by a puff of breath. I also set the intention of "as I extinguish the flame, the magic continues to be committed the next time I light the candle."

If you want to use the extinguishing of the flame as part of your spell, here are some interesting ways to add energy and drama.

Hard stop: When I am doing a cleansing, I will have the client hold a lit chime candle in each hand. When we are done, I have them quickly extinguish the candles, thus ending the cleansing. They do this quickly and with a hard wave down of the chime candles, thus putting them out. If the candles don't go out, I check to make sure the cleansing is complete.

Breathing in the essence: When I am manifesting something and it comes to pass before the candle is done, I will take a hard breath in to embody the energy and extinguish the candle. For safety's sake, be at least a foot away from the candle before you attempt to extinguish it in this way. If the candle doesn't go out, there is more to manifest, so let it burn until consumed.

Making that magic yours: During the course of your spell, you will probably need to extinguish the candle until you can attend it again. Blow it out with your breath and aspirate a little, anointing the candle with your essence—this dedicates the magic to you.

Reversing the flame: During reversing or clearing work, you can return the energy to the sender by turning the candle upside down and grounding the flame. You will spill wax when you do this, so take the appropriate precautions. You can ground the flame in dirt to send negative energy away from you and into the universal filter of Mother Earth. If you do this in nature, don't leave the wax remnants behind.

Temporary snuff: Gently snuffing a candle with a candle snuffer or another way to stop oxygen from getting to the flame is a gentle message that you are pausing the flame but the magic continues.

Drowning your sorrows: If a spell has gone in a way you do not want to continue, drown the flame in water and cleanse the candle of energy to stop its progression.

I'll say it again: never leave a burning candle unattended. Seriously, don't. Flame is unpredictable on its own, and when you add magic, it can get even weirder and more unpredictable. In my thirty-plus years of doing candle magic, I have watched flames jump and flare in unnatural ways. I have watched the heat of a flame shatter heatsafe glass. I have watched as the end of a candle burns down, the holder becomes extremely hot, creating scorch marks on the surface it is sitting on. The minute you think you know how your candle magic will work, it will change up on you. Taking chances with flame is just not worth the risk.

HOW MANY SPELLS CAN YOU DO AT ONCE?

One. Do one spell at a time. Doing multiple spells simultaneously will cross up your energy. You won't know what to vibrate: this spell or that spell. The one that is easiest to manifest will cancel out the other one, and you will need to start all over again. A laser-focused intent powers your spell faster than splitting your focus. Multitasking is a myth, especially in magic.

If you can't choose which spell to do, you have a deeper need that incorporates both. Redo the "Why Is That?" exercise and see what you can find.

But I Need to Fix Everything!

I understand that need. Now that you know better, you want to fix everything in your life at the same time. Just remember it took you years to get to this place of need, so it will take you a few years to heal and clear all the junk to manifest what you really want.

You will work on what is ready for evolution. Take your time, dig deep, and you won't have to rinse and repeat on the same issue too many times. You will revisit some issues as you work layer by layer to get to the core, but you will be spiraling through healing along the way.

WHEN NEW STUFF CROPS UP IN THE MIDDLE OF YOUR SPELL

Use your Candle Magic Journal to track the new issues that crop up during your spell. You may be experiencing what information needs to come to light, things you need to clear and heal, or who is interfering with your magic.

If something emerges, do the "Why Is That?" exercise to understand how it fits into the big picture of your spell and if you need to do something about it. Use your divination tools if you feel a little stuck—that's what they are there for.

THE ART OF
COCREATION

We don't create alone. We not only need each other to manifest our intention; we also actualize our magic in concert with all the divine energies in our universe. With the unique blend of ingredients that make up your spell, you are generating a vibration or signature of energy that will find its match in the divine. As they come together, all things are possible.

The goal of candle magic—or any magic for that matter—is to move your own limitations, fears, blocks, and beliefs out of the way so your intention can become real. As your magic manifests, it allows you to jump to the other side of your issue. When you make this leap, you can experience life without that limitation, which in turn grows the new belief that will heal this deficiency permanently. Imagine trying to muscle through that on your own, using your current energy and resources! The energy drain alone would cause you to give up before the finish line.

It takes two people to manifest your magic: you and the other person who flips the switch in your outer world. It takes two realms to manifest your magic as well: this physical one and the one in spirit. Building your relationships with the helpful spirits in your life, simply put, makes it easier. The closer the relationship with divine forces, the faster your magic manifests. Why? When you set up your spell, creating the vibration of what you want to manifest, it doesn't have to go searching the universe for a match. Instead, your divine allies fast track that match to you because they already know you and what need may be coming up in the future. A strong relationship with spirit will open the door for communication, allowing them to guide you to what they are already putting in play for you in the spirit world.

Set up the sacred space for your spirit guides and divine allies to support your magic, and then listen to their guidance through your candle burn and divination.

LIGHTS UPON THE ALTAR OF MAGIC

Growing up Catholic, my second favorite part of the mass was when the priest consecrated the altar. (My most favorite part was singing and maybe when it was over.) When I was studying Wicca, I loved the opening of the circle and calling in the elements and watchtowers. Participating in Santeria and Voodoo celebrations, I was enamored with the way any room was transformed into a place where the orisha and loa dwelled. I was filled with peace with the shamanic creation of sacred space. These traditions and more are proof to me that the divine exists, and creating an altar and sacred space illuminates their presence. With a sacred altar, I am honoring the work I am about to undertake, the energies I will be working with, and myself and my own sacredness. The many altars at Coventry keep me and my team attentive to the fact that we are doing sacred healing work in our building. Even spellwork I have done on the fly gets a moment of sacredness before launching.

Altars come in all shapes and sizes—from my lovely large wood buffet with my full-blown magical complements to my small rock that has been consecrated to be my portable sacred space. Slowing down to care for my altars and sacred spaces is one of my self-care activities. I know when I am caring for them, I am caring for my relationship with them.

Altars are where you connect to divine allies, interact with them, honor them, maintain your relationship with them, and feed them the energy needed to create change in the physical world. If you keep your altars energized and sacred, then any spell you put upon them gets a boost. When you take care of these spaces, they take care of you. Temporary sacred spaces can be quickly created with items you keep sacred on your altar. Simply place your consecrated items on any other surface, and sacred space is established. I remember when a very devout Christian conjure woman said that wherever you set your Bible is where God is. When she wanted to bless something, she set her Bible on it. I saw this in action during a class, and it shifted the vibration of a piece of cloth into a magical item buzzing with energy.

Before you start your candle spell, build your altar and consecrate your sacred space to transform it into a place where the divine can interact with your magic and bless what you are doing. Honor your magic efforts as a sacred moment; you deserve this amount of self-respect.

THE BASICS OF ALTAR SETUP

In its simplest form, an altar is a space that you have decided to make sacred and use to invite spirit into your life. It can be your car dashboard, the floor, a TV tray, a rock or tree stump, a spot in your garden, or even the exact place you are sitting or standing. To transform it from a regular old floor into a sacred space use these few simple steps to help you move from a regular person into a magical practitioner.

1. Breathe slowly for thirty breaths at a quarter of the speed of a normal breath. This will take about a minute, and that is the minimum amount of time it requires to move your brain into an alpha state and slow down the mental chatter.

2. Acknowledge the compass directions one by one, turning to face them. This gets your energy into the space, creates a container and boundary for your energy, and honors the caretaking spirits of the place.

3. Get grounded in this space. You can do this with a grounding visualization and also by stomping your feet as if you were rooting yourself or wiggling your toes into the ground to connect to its essence.

4. Cleanse the space. You can use a smudging technique with a variety of herbs and woods, sound vibration, light, energy visualization, or laughter. (Laughter does an amazing job at clearing energy.)

5. Invite your ancestors and divine allies to join you in this space as it is ready for them and the candle spell you are about to do.

TYPES OF ALTARS

I have about six altars at the Coventry factory. I will set up and take down special altars as needed, but my core altars are for ancestors, guides, guardians, prosperity, fairies/elementals, and my big magic altar. Temporary altars have been for communication, special goals, cooperation, staff attraction, healing, and mental health. I may have several candles going, but only one per altar. This many altars mean a lot of upkeep, offerings, and relationship building. For those who are beginning this journey of having a steady relationship with an altar, start simple and small; it's not a competition. I have this many altars because my divine allies asked for them and it gives me an excuse to get more magical flair.

You have the basics of setting up a working altar already at hand. Now before you follow my instructions on the type of altars you can create, check in with your own tradition or desired path. My altars are based on my Coventry Magic path and will probably differ from the traditions of someone reading this. I honor your path and tradition and wish for you to be as empowered in what you do, as I am empowered in what I do. Take what you learn here and make it your own.

Ancestor Altar

Your ancestors are the closest spirits to you. You are the culmination of their trials and tribulations, and they are completely vested in your success. In some ways they live within your DNA, no matter if you are in a direct lineage or adopted. When you marry into a family, their ancestors will always be yours, even after a divorce. I love to think about how the choices my ancestors made in their lives make my current life possible. My paternal grandfather made a choice to move to Toledo from Long Island, and my maternal grandfather moved his family from the Winnipeg, Manitoba, area in Canada to Detroit. If Baromeo Rochon had moved to Seattle like the rest of his family, my mother would have never met my father. I honor their choices, good or bad.

When you create an altar where you can connect with them, communicate, and ask for their blessings, you are honoring the struggle of your ancestors that got you here. If your ancestors were bastards that you never want to interact with, then you can use your ancestor altar to elevate their spirit, in turn healing the legacies you inherited from them. Even your bastard ancestors are interested in your success because they have left this mortal coil and are free from the limited perspective of the human form.

You can choose which ancestors you invite into your magical space. If no one in your known bloodline will fit the bill, call upon the unnamed ancestors that hold your spirit in high esteem; they will help you achieve your dreams and will empower your magic. When you invite them in, use the prayers they would be familiar with; you are honoring them, not trying to convert them. Even though they are well past the limitations of religion, your ancestors will see that you are honoring who they were.

In Santeria, I was taught to put the ancestor altar on the floor in the kitchen, bathroom, basement, or at the base of a tree. In reconstructionist magic, I was taught to put it by my front door. In the Buddhist tradition, ancestor altars are placed in the main living area on a high shelf. With all of these choices available, I listened to what my ancestors wanted, and they chose to be in my home office at my side. They wanted to be close to where my passion is. They wanted to have my back and work with me to fulfill my dreams. It is up to you where your ancestor altar makes sense, but I caution you not to put them in your bedroom. Your dreams will not allow you to rest, and you don't want them subjected to your hanky-panky—it's disrespectful.

Setting up your starter ancestor altar is easy. You need a white cloth to designate the space, pictures or something that resonates with their energy, flowers, a white candle, coffee, water, and something that they loved in life. Choose a place that you will see often but won't be disturbed by others. Lay out the cloth and arrange your items in a pleasing way. Knock on the altar or floor three times and call their names. Knock three times for each name you call to. Traditionally you would call them in order of the closest kin to you. It will go something like this:

"*Knock, knock, knock.* I call Betty Jo Jones-Phillips, daughter of Mary Louise Smith-Jones and Joseph Jones. *Knock, knock, knock.* I call to Mary Louise Smith-Jones, daughter of Mary and John Smith. *Knock, knock, knock.* I call to Joseph Jones, son of Sally and Robert Jones." Continue on with all the ancestors you want to call, including siblings, aunts, uncles, cousins. Then you knock nine times and call to the unnamed and unknown ancestors who help guide and bless your life.

Sit quietly for a bit to feel the shift in energy as your ancestors arrive. Show them this place as a spot to communicate with you and where you will leave them offerings. Tell them about the offerings you are leaving for them. You can use coffee to increase the clarity of communication, water to keep the channel open, flowers to give them energy to communicate with you, a candle to honor them and give them energy, and some of their favorite things to help them connect with you.

Say a prayer for them all, or more powerfully pray for each one of them. My ancestors are Catholic, and I find the Hail Mary is very well received. Sit quietly to feel or hear them. Talk to them out loud so they know this communication is intentional and not a random thought. Tell them about your life, your gratitude, and your struggles. Don't ask for anything yet.

It will take nine days of tending to your altar for your ancestors to become fully present. Replace the water and coffee every day, the flowers when they wilt, and if you leave any food, remove it after a few hours and bring new food every day. Relight the candle every time you tend your altar, letting it burn for a bit, and keep it in eyesight while it is burning.

After the nine days, bring your candle spells to your ancestor altar and ask for their blessing before you start the spell. Use the pendulum or coin method to get their answers. They may have something to add or change to make it better. Every time you do a spell, bring them an offering, flowers, food you have prepared, tobacco or their favorite brand of smokes, or a shot of their favorite spirits. You are asking them to affect your physical world, so give them the physical energy of your offerings to do so.

Tend to your ancestor altar regularly. They will tell you how often, but start weekly to keep them charged up. Flowers are not required every time, but bring something that has energy they can use, something that reminds them of the joy of life.

Purpose Altar

A purpose altar is created to keep a type of energy going in your life. Purpose altars can be for anything that is a regular issue—peace in the home, building a better relationship with your spouse, prosperity, creative energy, protection, guidance, health, etc. For instance, a prosperity altar I started for a specific goal was so successful, I couldn't bring myself to take it down. I decided to keep the prosperity in my life fed and active. I was learning how to move from a lack mindset to one of abundance, and this became a focal point that helped me on my journey. It grew from a candle, cloth, and spell paper to something filled with meaningful symbols that I share with my entire staff. I have shown them how to put their needs on the altar knowing that their abundance can also be abundance that I am able to share with them. I have created altars in my home to keep it clear as I struggled with a relationship issue. I had one in my kitchen for healthy choices. Right now I have one on my desk for writing that will be dismantled and blessed when I am done with this book.

Start with the basics on your altar: clean and cleanse the space, place a cloth or something that gives the altar a boundary, energize the space, invite in your divine allies to bless it, and then set your candle spell. Make this space visually appealing for you, and add things that bring you joy and energy to your goal. Have fun! If you are doing it right, magic is fun and appeals to the inner child that powers up your intention and magical energy.

Energizing your purpose altar can be done with stones, spirits, waters, incense, flame, sound, and so on. Wake up the energy in this space by knocking on it and calling it into being. Spray it with a little Florida Water to give it a boost, and then give it a party with your other items. The only limit is your imagination. Put stones in the four directions, mouth-spray alcohol (similar to a spit take), play your favorite/appropriate music, chant, ring bells, drum. Bring your personality in and have a blast.

Once you get this altar set up, do a bit of divination to see if it is ready for your spell. Pendulums work well with this as you can read the energy of the space with how wide and fast the pendulum is rotating and in what direction. Get quiet and listen to your divine allies and their guidance. I got a really cool stone that I wanted on my prosperity altar, but my guides said no way. They did this by getting me to knock it over, break things with it, and more. Looking deeper, the stone's energy was too clearing—I wanted to keep the money, not clear it all out.

Nature Altars

Truth be told, I am not an expert at creating nature altars. Between allergies, sun sensitivity, and bugs, being out in nature is not my first thought for my magic, nor my happy place. Because of this, I went to my witch sister Susan Diamond of Serpent's Kiss in Santa Cruz, California, to talk about how she creates amazing experiences out in nature. From her Witches in the Woods events to her SeaSide Sorcery experience, building temporary altars in nature is her area of expertise.

Nature altars are used to tap into powerful elemental and primal energies to power up your spell. Using the tide to bring something into your life or take it out, a natural crossroads to change the course of something, or a rotting stump to eliminate something or reverse a curse, Susan will build a quick temporary altar within the rhythm of the natural space to honor the elementals and do her candle spell.

Since this is a candle magic book and candles have flames, let's be clear: do not light a candle in a wildfire-prone area! Actually, be very careful of any flame or heat you bring into nature, with incense, smudging, candles, burning tobacco, etc. You can always charge up an unlit candle in nature and finish the spell at home. This lines up with Susan's main rule for nature altars: do no harm. Do not leave things in nature that will harm the environment, including putting it at risk with flame. The elemental and primal energies you are working with would definitely get irritated and could flip your spell on you. Go ahead and do your candle spell in nature if conditions allow it, but if you burn a candle, take the remnants of the wax away with you or finish the burn at home. If your spell involves you leaving something behind, make sure it is biodegradable. This brings to mind some old conjure tricks that involve nuts, mercury, and wax that are supposed to be thrown into a moving body of water. Don't do that. Modernize those spells with safer materials or do something else. Treat nature as a beloved partner, and it will bless your magic.

Setting up a nature altar involves connecting to the spirits of the area and asking permission, honoring the spirits, inviting them to bless and assist the spell, and then doing your work. Work with the landscape and ask to be shown the perfect place to work your magic. Be still and listen, and you will find that place. If you are in the depths of nature, there is no need for clearing or energizing: flow with the energy there and tap into it with respect. If you come to an area that needs energetic clearing and energizing, do the healing work for the space, but do not cast a spell there. When we are tuned in to our magical self, the elementals call to us to heal where needed before we do our spell. That energy is always a blessing to your spell.

Garden Altars

Again, this is not my wheelhouse. (I'm more of a rock garden kind of gal.) I do, however, have big envy of the amazing altars I have been honored to see and work in. To give this subject the honor it deserves, I turned to the ultimate garden witch, Ellen Dugan. When I asked her for input, she was out in her garden with her granddaughter, passing on the magical tradition. I was talking to the correct witch. In Ellen's *Garden Witchery* and *Garden Witch's Herbal*, she takes you through all the ways you can make your garden magical.

Ellen's advice for setting up a garden altar is to find a spot in your garden that welcomes your altar and start there. The more magic you do in this spot, the more magically powerful it will get. You can gradually place stones, statues, water elements, and plants that will enhance your altar. Sacred spaces in your garden can be years in the making, so don't be in a rush to have it perfect. Creating a garden altar is a magical journey of discovery and awakening. It can also be your secret. This space does not need to scream magic; it can look like every other spot and still be sacred to you. If you are in the city or suburbs, there will be someone blowing their leaves, kids playing, or a dog barking when you go out to do your magic. It's OK, you already made this place sacred, and when you sink into it, all the other noise will fall away.

You don't need a big yard for a garden altar. You can do this with a container garden on your patio or even a window garden. Don't let space stop you from bringing nature into your magic. Ellen spoke of a city witch friend of hers who could take any random item as a planter and turn an entire room into her garden, letting her window garden spill into her entire space. That too is a garden altar. Have fun with this! Let the joy of spellcrafting spill into any space you use.

Big Magic Altars

If you choose to have a big magic altar, this will be a sacred space that anchors your magic and honors your spirit guides and divine allies. Different from a purpose altar that has a specific focus, your big magic altar is where you go for your day-to-day magical needs, and it will keep you and your spell energized. My big magic altar represents spiritual muscle memory that will transport me right into the alpha brain state where magic happens. I set up my altar to immediately create a sacred space around me when I approach and honor it. My altar was created over decades and has been housed on different furniture pieces and decorated with a rotating cast of items, proving that the altar transcends the physical.

I started my big magic altar shortly after Coventry was born. It began on my desk, moved to an overhead shelf, shifted to the lobby, came back to my desk, went onto its own credenza, came back to a shelf, and now it's on a big buffet credenza that also stores my magical supplies. Through each incarnation, I cleansed the space, charged it up, invited in my spiritual court, and carefully arranged my altar items. The ceremony is my own and has evolved over time with the basic elements changing to support my needs of the moment.

Setting Up a Big Magic Altar

1. Start with the same rhythm for a purpose altar, and add a few more things in.

2. Cleanse the space and add specific altar cloths.

    a. Start with a black or dark brown cloth to represent the earth.

    b. Create white backdrop in some way to represent the divine. It can be a white wall, a tall white item, a white ceiling, or a white cloth tacked onto the wall.

    c. Place a red cloth on top of the black/brown one to represent the quickening that comes from connecting heaven and earth.

3. Energize the altar by inviting in each cardinal compass direction and anchoring it to the earth in some way. Large rocks beneath the altar, a natural walking stick or staff that leans on the altar, a railroad spike tied to each leg of the altar are some of the ways to anchor the directions.

4. Invite in your spiritual court with conversation, prayers, and one candle lit on the center of the altar. As you sense their arrival, start to place their items on the altar. (This is where the altar items can rotate. Some don't fit your energy anymore and are making room for what is next.)

5. Cast a blessing spell as soon as the altar is set, and then return to your daily magical practice.

The big magic altar ceremony evolved as my spiritual knowledge and spiritual court grew. Each action is in honor of a tradition I have been trained in, and before I incorporated any new spirit or ceremony, I checked with my spiritual court for acceptance. I knew that some of my guides needed their own dedicated altar because they didn't vibe with my big magic altar.

I encourage you to create your own altar if you don't have one already. You can start small—a wood box from the craft store is an easy base. Setting up that altar for your spell will become a ceremony in itself, transporting you to a magical state. It can also double as your magical toolbox, allowing you to keep your altar away from prying eyes and inquisitive minds. As you grow your big magic altar, you will find that your magical results grow too. You are nurturing the belief in your own spellcasting ability, growing your relationship and trust in your spiritual court, and together that creates the kind of positive spark that brings big magic.

An anchored big magic altar can be projected into other spaces. *What!?* I know, right: it blew my mind too! When I did my first teaching tour in 2007, I tested this theory. I was in a new space every other day. I didn't know what

I would be walking into, and I was teaching big concepts and asking people to get vulnerable. What if the space had unhealthy energy? I didn't have the room to bring the whole shebang with me, so I created an energetic construct that was anchored on my altar. For me this was the tree of life. I could quickly visualize the tree expanding from the center of the room to encompass the whole space. I added a stone in each direction to anchor it in place, and I was ready to teach.

This theory was tested and proven at a convention when my class ended up being right after a demonology class and who knows what other classes before that. It was a busy room to say the least. I pulled on my big magic altar and transported the sacred space within moments. The energy that was in that room was pushed out, and I had a powerful class where my students got vulnerable and unlocked their own big magic. If I had had to clear the room in a conventional way, it would have been a struggle and I would have changed my class plan from experiential to theory only.

Divinity Altars

Remember when I said some of my divine allies were not compatible with the spiritual court on my big magic altar? They get their own space that I have to ensure is attended to. I try to limit the number of altars I have to keep, as they are a commitment in energy and time. Also there are specific

---

Warning from your Aunt Jacki: If you take on an altar, don't let it go fallow. If you build an altar and then ignore it, let it get dusty and dirty, and start using it to store junk, your magic will become impotent. An active altar stays connected to you and your energy. When you don't care for your magical spaces, they become a drain on you. Think about it this way: When you run your lights and radio in your car, you drain the battery. To recharge it, you need to start it up and drive it around to spin up your alternator. Your spells are the alternator to the battery of your altar. You are the altar-nator; keep your magical space charged and ready for your next candle spell and you will pack a bigger magical punch. My six altars need me to keep their batteries charged, and in turn they keep me charged up too. It's a lot of work—and totally worth it. When you are done with an altar, thank the spirits, release them from your call, and cleanse all of your items.

THE BIG BOOK OF CANDLE MAGIC

prescriptions for many divinity altars preventing me from creating a generic how-to for you to follow. If you are called by a divine being to create a space for them, get instructions from a devotee if you can. At the very least, do your research before you agree to work with them. I was called by Grand Bois, a nature/elemental loa from Haitian Voudon before a prosperity class I went to. Grand Bois, meaning "big wood," was in my dreams the night before as a man in a tree. He wanted to come home with me. The teacher, a Voudon priest, invoked him for the ritual in the class, and so I understood who was in my dream. Before I said yes to coming home, I negotiated the relationship. We settled on a twelve-month stay as I was working through something he could help with.

It is easy to culturally appropriate rich traditions from around the world. The way to ensure that you are practicing cultural appreciation instead is to do your research, connect with a devotee or follower, and honor the divine being in a way that aligns with their original culture. Educate yourself on the culture or origin for this divine ally and understand their struggle so you may be an ally in return.

CANDLE MAGIC IN ACTION

LIGHTING THE CANDLE

When you are lighting the candle, you are quickening your magic. You are the alchemist adding the final element that will transform your idea into reality. My feelings about the final lighting of the candle remind me of the memes from the 2010s: what you think you are doing, what others think you are doing, and what you are really doing.

What we think we are doing is taking a rush wick (as used in the Middle Ages), lighting it from the hearth fire, and gently touching it to our candle to make a sacred flame. What others think we are doing is creating a flame with our magic powers. What we are really doing is getting that candle lit, and we can't find our matches . . .

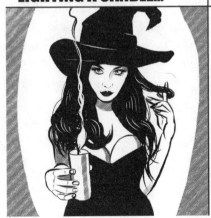 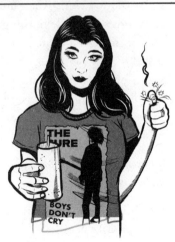

In my head, I will always be witch #1.

A box of utility matches can be your prized magical tool. They usually come in a pack of three, they light easily, and darnit, they feel magical. Many witches feel that this is the only way to light a candle spell as lighters are too gauche and a match feels so natural and in sync with their spell. A good solid lighter from the gas station may save your spell from never happening when you can't find those matches, however. Match, lighter, taper, rush—you can make any of these items purposeful and magical.

When you light the candle, you are giving energy you collected for this spell permission to go forth and manifest. Say your incantation, restate your goal, and spend time talking to the candle and visualizing what your life will be like after your spell is a success.

NEVER LEAVE A BURNING CANDLE UNATTENDED—THAT MEANS YOU!

I'm not kidding, and this is why this very serious statement gets its own spot in the table of contents. *Do not leave your candle lit when you are not there!*

Candle = fire

Fire = unpredictable

Unpredictable fire = tragedy

In case you are thinking I'm talking to someone else, *NO*, I am talking to you. In our 21st-century world, there are so many distractions you can quickly forget that you have a candle burning somewhere outside your eyeshot. I know hundreds of stories about near and total tragedy occurring when a candle is unattended.

Earlier, on page 138, I shared a few different ways to extinguish your candle while maintaining the integrity of your spell. It is so simple that if you overthink it, you will confuse yourself. You can always use this prayer for extinguishing your candle temporarily:

> *As I extinguish your flame, your magic continues, to be refreshed when I light you again.*

That's it. This prayer, or a variation on it, has worked for my own candle spells for over three decades. I have proven this model. Your magic has begun, you have given it purpose, and it is working for you. The flame renews and refreshes it, but it isn't a deal breaker if you temporarily put it out. Extinguishing a candle will not kill the spell unless you declare it so.

Also please, for the love of magic, remove all packaging from your non-container candle before you light it. The label, plastic, box, and any other packaging are never meant to remain on the candle as it burns. No matter how perfect it looks, it's packaging and flammable.

HOW THE CANDLE BURNS

Ceromancy is the spiritual language of candles. It starts with the halo of spirit around your flame. This halo represents the divine influence of your spell. It is what you focus on when you want to communicate with spirit to gain a deeper understanding of your candle spell and its manifestation. Spirit, in turn, talks to you through how the candle burns. The flame, the smoke, the wax, and the soot are part of this language.

The more candle spells you have under your belt, the clearer your understanding of this divination system. The flicker of the flame tells of the energy in play, the lifting smoke tells of what you are releasing, the drip of the wax what you are manifesting, and the soot what you overcame. Each candle you burn in your spell will react in a unique way—which is why you never leave them unattended. Your intent, need, and ingredients will influence how your candle will burn. This is your personal ceromancy, and your candle spells will talk to you and defy standard candle readings. For one person, a fast burn will mean that there was no substance to the spell. For another, a fast-burning candle will mean that they *needed* this spell and it will manifest with speed.

Grab your Candle Magic Journal and record how your candle burns, what it is telling you, and then the results of that spell over time. Tarot readers learn the personalities of their decks in the same way; they pull a card and record what happens in their day. The same applies to learning the language of candles for yourself.

Things That Will Affect Your Candle Burn

Before you start interpreting your candle, some candle magic debunking is in order. It's exciting to see a big change in your candle, only to discover a big old draft is fanning the flame. Check for the mundane before you start on the mystical.

Drafts will cause your flame to flicker, get larger, and give off more smoke. Every time your flame flickers, it releases a puff of smoke that creates soot. Drafts also cause one side of your candle to burn faster than another.

Wicks cut too short will cause your candle to go out. There isn't enough room for the wick to pull up the wax and burn it off. The advice to trim your wick to a quarter inch is not always sound. Wider candles, slower-burning candles, candles with stuff in them may need more of a wick. I start with one inch, and the wick naturally burns down and settles to its optimal height.

Wicks that are not centered during manufacturing will cause your candle to burn to one side, drip more, and possibly go out. Uncentered wicks can also happen when you extinguish them between burn times. After extinguishing your candle, use a tool to lift the wick so it cools in the right place.

Heavily dressed candles can cause a faster burn or clog the wick. Flowers in wax are so lovely—and so dangerous. Finely ground herbs will sink to the bottom of the melting wax as you burn the candle, but some flowers float and get pulled toward the wick, risking a candle bonfire. Finely ground herbs can get wicked up and gutter the flame. If your wick is clogged with herbs and glitter, candle surgery is needed to finish the burn. Crystals in your wax can fall against the flame and crack, even projecting pieces away from the candle. They can also fall over and put the flame out.

Look for the technical difficulties before interpreting your spell. Then again, you can also look at it as destiny. You picked or were sent that candle for a reason, and maybe that is part of the message.

Reading the Flame

Strong, Steady Flame

A strong, steady flame represents power and energy for your spell. You can take it as a sign that your magic is working quickly and effectively. If the flame is extraordinarily high, that may mean that the energy of the spell is going too fast and may burn out too quickly with results that don't last. Spiritual cleansing or banishing candle spells with a high flame show that a lot is being burned off.

With a figure candle, a strong flame can mean several things. The person that candle represents may be winning or angry, or they may be doing their own spell to manipulate the situation. It can also mean that the decision is in their hands and they are in charge. When two figure candles are used, the higher and stronger flame shows you who is dominant in the situation—who will affect the outcome more. If that is not what you want, you may need to adjust your spell.

Weak Flame

A weak or small flame represents your magic working really hard to get through a tough block. That block may be someone working against you, or it may be your own junk getting in your way. A slightly smaller than average flame tells you that this spell will need a lot of hard work to manifest. If your candle has a very small flame, check to make sure you didn't trim it too short. If you did, pour some molten wax out, making the wick longer. (You may need some candle surgery here.) Then do some spiritual cleansing work

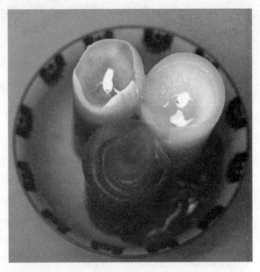

For this candle spell to draw a love interest, the candle that was snuffed by the wax drips represented the love interest. Message: They are not interested in you; move on.

while the candle is burning. Use the size of the flame as a barometer for the effectiveness of your spiritual cleansing. If the flame never gets larger or goes back to being small, extinguish the candle and investigate a different direction to attaining your magical goal. If you keep trying to dig the wick out, you will just end up breaking it off—and a wickless candle is just useless!

Flame Goes Out during Spell

Put your spell aside if the flame goes out on its own, and do a spiritual cleansing. This is a big block or outside interference. Cleanse yourself and your environment thoroughly and ask for assistance to help you clear what you cannot sense. Van Van is an excellent remedy to use as it will also clear out any work being done against you. Also do a "Why Is That?" reading to find out what is going on with your spell.

Flickering Flame

If you have a flickering flame, first check for any draft, including people moving in and out of the room. Once that is settled, you could be getting a message that there are spirits present, which can be confirmed with a pendulum. If your spirits want to communicate with you in this way, give them their own candle to talk to you and play with. Another message may be that the candle is burning off the bad wishes of others. That may not be interfering with your spell yet, but you can light a reversing or protection candle to make sure it never does.

Tips from your Aunt Jacki: Don't assume you have a bad candle if your wick goes out. I was testing our new candleholders with my company's Protection and Stability candles because they were handy. The candle kept going out. When I tested lighter color candles, I didn't have the same issue, and I was confused about why only the dark candles did that. It took me a minute and having others test the candles to realize that this was a message to me. I was being worked on by someone. I took care of that situation, and now those candles burn just fine.

Jumping Flame

Flickering flames are gentle. Jumping flames are aggressive and a sign of anger in love spells. They can also be seen as bursts of energy, so look for some immediate results in your spell. If you get the jumping flame in the beginning of your spell (and it is not a love spell), you are off to a decent start; if it never calms down, consider whom this spell may be angering.

If you are using two figure candles, your message is that there is anger between the two: pay attention to which flame is jumping. Add some lavender or other soothing fragrances to your candle spell to calm any heated, angry energetic discussions.

Sparks from the Candle

If your candle sparks, first look for hot embers on the table and floor. Magically, a spark from the candle means that your wish is being fulfilled. To avoid the bad sparks that may burn holes in things, make sure to trim off the carbon balls that collect on the end of the wick.

Flame Pointing in a Specific Direction

A flame bending in a certain direction may either relate to the compass direction your energy is heading or coming from or may be a message from an elemental. Check your compass and pay attention to the direction.

North: It may be a long journey, but your spell is definitely manifesting.

East: Look for ideas that will solve your problem; if they are not here now, they will be arriving soon.

South: You are going to have to work through some anger, you will be filled with passion, or you may get a burst of energy to make things happen.

West: You may get very frustrated and emotional over this spell before it manifests. Make time for a good cry and be sure to nurture your spell a bit more to coax it along.

Fast or Slow Burn

In the spirit of never leaving a burning candle unattended, pay attention to how slow or fast yours burns. If your spell suddenly takes off while you are paying attention, you will avoid falling flames, dripping wax, personal damages, and "oh, shit!" moments.

Candle safety lessons from your Aunt Jacki: For an intense spiritual cleansing spell, I placed my candle in a tempered glass holder. I knew I was going to be working in the factory and would not be in my office to attend it, so I overprotected. I placed the candleholder in a cake pan filled with sand, on a cookie sheet on my altar. It wasn't long before the candleholder exploded, the wax absorbed into the sand, and the flame lit the sand into a million wicks. The hot sand popped and crackled and spit flame all over my altar, and the whole thing caught on fire! Someone happened to be putting mail on my desk and found the fire before it became an inferno! They yelled *FIRE* in a candle factory and brought me running from the next room, only fifteen feet away. Yes, I broke big energetic ties with that spell, and we were lucky enough to put it out before major damage happened. Keep your candles close and in your line of sight, and watch what the burn tells you about your spell.

Candleholder Cracks or Explodes

Candleholders that have a crack, are too thin, are overused and never cleaned, or have the flame leaning against the glass will crack and potentially explode. When they explode, the glass gets pushed away from the center. If that wasn't the case in your cracking candleholder, you have a protection issue or you broke through a big block. (See story above.) Refer to your favorite divination tool to see if someone is attacking you. If this was a reversing candle, then you have big trouble in Little China, and it's time to pull out bigger magical guns.

Candle Does Not Burn or Burns Very Slowly

Reference Weak Flame above.

Flame Tunnels Down the Center

A candle that is tunneling down the center can also split. Check the wick as it may be too small for the candle, or you may not be burning it for a long enough period of time before extinguishing it (one hour per inch of diameter). If that is not the case, you are dealing with an internal process, and you need to conquer some fears before you will achieve success. If the candle splits down the middle, you are not decided on what you want.

Candle Burns to One Side

The first thing to check is the position of the wick and for a draft. If the wick is not centered, it will burn to one side. If the wick is centered and the air still, you need to look at your spell: Is it one-sided? Are you looking at this from the wrong perspective? This can also mean that your spell will be only partially effective or you are using the wrong candle spell. The one-sided burn could also mean that there is more interference from one area in your life.

Candle Has More Than One Flame

Multiple flames can be caused by soot balls from the wick falling into the wax, herbs you put in the candle catching on fire, or the candle accidently having two wicks. The wick splitting can cause a double flame; the flame splitting on the wick on its own is the most uncommon phenomenon. If this is not a technical difficulty, the meaning of this double flame can be really good or really bad. The energy is either coming from two places or being cut in half. In protections or hexing spells, it means that the intended target is aware of what you are doing and is sending the energy back to you.

Candle's Entire Top Is on Fire

This is generally caused by candles that have been heavily dressed with lots of herbs on top. Be aware of this potential fire hazard when dressing your candle. In a magical sense, when you have a reasonable amount of herbs on your dressed candle and it all goes up in flame, that means your magic is on hyperspeed. If this is for a controlling spell, a massive flame means that spirits are guarding the person you are trying to control. For protection spells, that means spirits are protecting you and someone is trying to get at you.

Candle Burns Down Quickly

Some burning candles have a large flame, sending the message that your spell is strong and effective and you will be manifesting your goal soon. Upon occasion, regular- to small-size flames will have a quick-burning candle, creating an even more powerful portent telling you that you needed this energy, and you needed it fast. When candles go quickly, take it as a sign to burn another candle for the same cause.

Candle Burns Slowly

Slow-burning candles and small flames go hand in hand. Refer to the weak flame definition above. If you have a slow-burning candle and a regular flame, the candle is doing its job and getting you through the hard parts. Do not mess with the candle to make it burn faster; let the magic work.

READING THE WAX

In the Witches Union Spell Casters Club Facebook group, the most asked question is, "What do you see in my candle wax?" The shapes that dripping wax makes are fascinating to watch and mystic in the messages they may be giving you. But this could also be just heat and gravity with no message at all. How can you tell the difference between a message and a mess? Outside of spilling the wax for a reading, you discern the message of your candle through your own intuition. You will want to ground, center, and open up to hearing your divine allies and the message they have for you.

Candle Wax Reading Exercise

Start with your favorite grounding and centering technique. If you don't have one, sit still in a comfortable position, focus on the flame of the candle, and let your vision get soft. Breathe slowly and steadily, allowing your frantic thoughts to unwind, your stress to release, and your senses to relax from their constant alert status.

When you are at a place of calm and ease, allow your psychic senses to open. Visualize your third eye opening and allow a sixth sense to take over for the other five.

Story from your Aunt Jacki: I was lighting an ancestor candle for my sister who was going through a rough time. It was set up perfectly to not spill over my shelf and onto my printer, yet in the unpredictable way of the flame and candle, it spilled anyway. It did it the moment I went to the bathroom. When I got back, I saw a clear wax figure of someone looking over the candleholder into the candle. My ancestors were watching over her. Around the same time as my message, she sent a picture of the candle spell she was doing in her home and there was an angel in the wax. Thanks, ancestors! Message received.

Gently move your gaze from the candle flame to the wax drips. Follow the pattern and allow your imagination to take charge. Think of the times as a child when you watched the clouds in the sky change form and become familiar shapes. If you looked too hard, the shape disappeared. Keep your gaze soft, filled with childlike imagination and belief in magic. Turn the candle and holder if needed and look at it from a new perspective. Write down your observations without judgment or thought. Let the words flow from your psychic centers. When you are done writing, take a deep breath and come back to the room.

To get back into your body, wiggle your toes, clap your hands, and, if needed, gently touch your forehead to close your psychic center.

Reread what you wrote and connect it to your original intent, "Why Is That?" worksheet, and words of power. Is there a message or connection? Write this in your Candle Magic Journal.

You may not get a message, and there is nothing wrong if you don't. The candle and spell are doing their job and there may be nothing to report. If you are not satisfied, use your favorite divination tool or spill some wax (described below) to check in.

If you get a message and see symbols in your wax, let go of any book definition of those symbols and ask yourself what they have to do with your spell. Start with a literal meaning and let it become a personal definition.

In the back of this book is a simple symbol-meaning index. Remember to use this as a guide and make the symbols personal and focused on your candle spell.

EXTRA DIVINATION DURING YOUR SPELL

Another layer to candle divination is purposeful reading of the wax and smoke. This is so fun and worth experimenting on. Your candle spell may be acting right and doing its job, but you just *have to* know what's going on! This is also a specialized reading technique that brings a unique new insight.

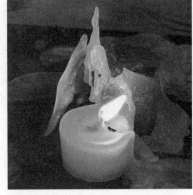

Do you see the angel? This was a candle spell asking for support.

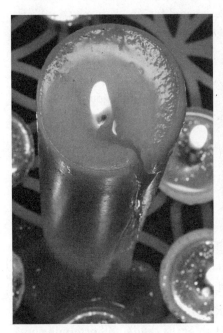

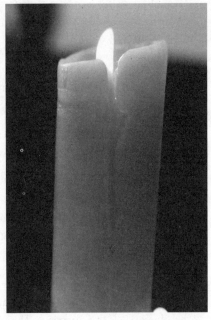

In this candle spell for personal development, the crack that developed showed there was a breakthrough.

There are two ways you can divine what is happening during your spell: (1) pouring molten wax in cold water, and (2) running paper over the flame to capture symbols from the smoke.

Use your favorite grounding and centering method or the one described in Candle Wax Reading Exercise to get in the space to do some divination.

Spilling Wax

Candle wax readings can be compared to tea leaf reading. The symbology is the same, you are using a cup/bowl shape, and if you want to take it further, you can divide the bowl into twelve pie-slice–shaped sections to represent the twelve houses in astrology or the twelve months of the year like they do in tea leaf readings.

To spill your wax for divination purposes, you will need a black or a clear bowl filled with four cups of water (or one liter for my metric friends), something to mark the starting point, and a candle. I would suggest doing this on a towel to soak up any spills—I guarantee you will have some.

If you are using a candle already designated for a spell, bring your bowl over to the candle. You don't want to disturb the molten wax until you are ready to divine.

For a new candle, dress and light your candle about thirty minutes before you plan on doing a reading as you will want a good amount of molten wax to pool around the wick.

Dress your candle using a divination, psychic powers, or spirit communication oil and anoint it top down. White candles are easier to read with as you can see the interesting shapes and shadows in the wax more easily.

Magically charge your bowl of water with three drops of the same oil with which you anointed the candle. Get in touch with your inner witch, open your psychic centers, and prepare to divine some wax.

How you drip the wax into the water is a bit of trial and error to master the technique. It is best to let the molten wax flow from the lit candle while you ask the question. The width of the candle will determine how much molten wax is available to use with each tip of the candle. Drip-less tapers, utility, and chime candles just don't work for candle divination. You need a pool of wax to get a readable shape, and you don't get that from those very efficient candles. You also want a candle that is not too far down into the holder, or most of your wax will end up on the side of the holder. Find your patience and let the candle get a nice pool of wax rather than a few drips. It's the pool of wax that will actually make the symbol you are going to divine; a drip gives you nothing but a dot. Wax will move in the water and will continue to float around during the reading, giving you an interesting interaction between drips of wax. You can even use different colors of wax for different questions. If you are using the same candle for all of the wax readings, you will need to wait between questions for the molten wax to collect again.

Every divination system needs a get-to-know-you stage, including wax readings. As you explore this system, start by asking questions you know the answers to. This will get you in tune with how the wax divination will work for you. Look at the symbols, where they float to, and how they relate to each other. Start with your own intuition and experience before looking at the symbol list in the index.

Using a clear bowl for your wax divination allows you to place an astrological chart underneath the bowl to give you a quick reference as to what house or part of the querent's life the symbol floats toward. The closer to the center, the further away the issue is (or the further in the past); the closer to the edge of the bowl, the closer it is to arriving.

Once you read the wax in the bowl and it is fully cooled, pick it up. The bottom of the wax dripping will hold even more symbols and interesting messages. Wax reading is very three-dimensional!

Refer to the symbols index in the back of the book for more insight into your ceromancy reading.

Reading the Smoke

Welcome to the world of capnomancy and libanomancy. Capnomancy is smoke divination and libanomancy is divination of incense smoke. The portents for this type of divination are simple. A thin, straight plume of smoke is a good sign. Large puffs of smoke are considered a bad omen, and if the smoke touches the ground, you are in trouble and you need to take immediate action. The direction in which the smoke travels is also very telling.

Seeing smoke at all is communicating to you: (a) the fragrance in the candle is burning, or (b) pay attention. This is not like a campfire; the smoke doesn't just follow you.

Toward You

If the smoke travels toward you, congratulations, your spell is a success, and you will get what you want.

Away from You

If the smoke is traveling away from you, it means that your spell will take more time than you think to manifest.

The Candle Smokes Heavily and Turns the Glass Black

First, check the length of the wick; when it is too long, it will smoke. Second, check for drafts; air currents that move the flame will cause puffs of smoke. Also, if this is a poor-quality scented candle, it will smoke more than a higher-quality candle. If this is not the case, you have someone sending you the whammy, and it may be interfering with your spell. If the flame is strong and smokin', you are burning off negativity. If this happens while using a controlling spell, that spell may be turned back upon you. Remember, every scented candle will soot to some degree.

The Smoke Travels in a Specific Direction

Northbound smoke tells you that you have more work to do. Success will not be easy or right away, but it will come. For issues of health, this is not a good sign, and you need to seek medical attention.

Eastbound smoke tells you that you need to make a few adjustments, but that you will manifest your spell in the end.

Southbound smoke is telling you that things are happening fast. If this is a health spell, it means that you are recovering and will get better soon.

Westbound smoke means you are not emotionally balanced about this situation and you need to step back or you will mess things up more. Take a moment to do the "Why Is That?" exercise to uncover what your deeper need is for this situation.

Smoke Reading on Your Spell

I also do a type of smoke divination with a note card and candle. Using the candle in your spell, you will be intercepting the smoke with the note card and then reading the patterns that appear. Your first impression of the image the smoke made is the most important part of the message. It is best to relax your mind and sink into a bit of meditation before you do this or any divination. Don't judge what you see; just understand that the message is simply a message. Your power lies in what you do with the message.

Gather a candle (or use the candle in your spell), clean note card, and a bowl of water for safety. The thicker the paper, the better. You don't want the paper drooping into the flames and catching fire!

Start by thinking of a question. Hold the card on the opposite edges, then move the card in irregular patterns directly over, but not into, the flame. You need to move at a moderately quick pace so the paper does not catch on fire—thus the bowl of water for safety. Don't move too fast as the smoke should have time to make an impression on the paper. Move the paper as you are speaking your question out loud. This will take twenty to thirty seconds tops. Flip the card over and see what images you find. The position of the image has no bearing; only the image itself does.

Use your intuition to tell you what this means, but if you get stuck, look at the symbols index in the back of the book.

If you want to ritualize this a bit more, start by writing on the paper with lemon juice (a paintbrush works perfectly for this). Write the name of the person you are interested in, the problem you are facing, or the wish you want fulfilled. You won't be able to see what you are writing, but you will once you put heat to it. After the lemon dries, run the paper over the flame in the same way as above. Look at where your symbol lands in relation to the words that appeared from the heat of the flame. The layering of these two actions gives you a very interesting reading.

DISPOSING OF WAX AND SPELL REMAINS

"It ain't over till it's over."

—*Yogi Berra*

Your spell is not complete until you dispose of the remains. You will want to complete the clearing or anchor what you are bringing to you. Leaving this undone is like leaving money on the table or a baseball inning unplayed. At the very least, for spells that bring increase, love, or healing, thank your ingredients for their work, release the energy, cleanse the tools, and dispose of the remains in your garbage. For spells that are clearing something from you, take all the remains, place them in a garbage bag without touching them, and throw it away in a garbage can or dumpster not connected to you in any way.

You can also use the remains to anchor the magic you did into your life, start another spell, or make a work of art. Below are some ideas on how to get creative with the end of your spell.

Prosperity

Make money symbols for your prosperity altar. Carry prosperity wax with you in a mojo bag. Use the wax to anoint a contract or "lucky" money. Create a perpetual prosperity candle by burning each candle in the same large (supersized) candleholder, letting the drips remain.

Protection

Use the remnants as an anchor in your yard or a potted plant near your front door. Take biodegradable remains to the grave of an ancestor with an offering and request for continual protection. If you can't get to a grave, use the base of a tree that you visit often.

Love

Make wax hearts for love and put them in a sweet jar for your love. Use the remains in your lingerie drawer. Create a mojo bag that you keep with you.

Clearing

Get rid of it. Don't keep any clearing remains.

Healing

Put the wax in a poppet or doll to promote healing in the body.

HOW LONG WILL IT TAKE FOR MY SPELL TO WORK?

"It depends" is not the answer you are looking for, but it is the only answer anyone can give. The speed of your spell manifesting is driven by several things: the momentum of your life to align with the spell, the complexity of your magical ask, and how much clearing/healing you need to open the road for your spell to become reality.

If you are already moving in the direction of your spell, it will manifest faster. There is an abundance of energy that aligns with the end goal of your spell and you are open to it becoming a part of your life. If your spell is very different from the life you are currently living, it will take longer to actualize. There are many issues that you will need to heal and evolve for your spell to have a foundation to manifest on.

The better question is, "How can I tell if my spell is working?" Tracking your spell and the small changes that happen every day in your Candle Magic Journal will show you the slow, steady progress and keep you in gratitude. Slipping into fear or doubt is a perfect way to sabotage your spell.

Your spell is working for you even if you don't get what you want. Look for the message about what is in your way or what needs to change. Every time I do a big goal-setting session at Coventry and back it up with magic, something falls apart. At first I thought this was my magic breaking to someone working against me when it was really the universe getting things out of my way to assist me in making my goals happen. People would quit, something would break, sales would suddenly slow down, or a whole list of other mini disasters. I started looking at this as my energy and life shaking out what was going to keep me down. Be nimble, be flexible, go with the flow, and pay attention to the message around you.

HOW SOON DO I CAST AGAIN?

Did you get what you wanted? No need to cast again. Are you waiting for your spell to work? Do a reading with your favorite divination tool to see if your spell is still working but just taking a long time.

If you are feeling the need to back your spell up with another one, most likely what's really required is a clearing before you do another spell. There are expectations, hooks into your energy, or fear blocks that are preventing your spell from manifesting.

CANDLE MAGIC JOURNALING

Before you read this section, go get that pretty blank journal you have on the shelf. You are going to use it now—you deserve to put your candle spells in something special. If not that blank journal, grab a spiral notebook because you are starting your Candle Magic Journal right now. This isn't your grimoire where you record your magic for all of posterity, this is journal of experiments and observations on your candle spells. You may not keep up with it regularly and no one is mad about that. Just start it today. Make it messy. Make it magical. Make it yours.

Open your journal, flip three pages, and start numbering your pages. This will come in handy when you start creating your index of your candle spells later on. Get zen about this step and let your mind float as you number your pages. This is part of the commitment to returning to your Candle Magic Journal when you do your spells.

The next several pages are your worksheet templates to build and record your spell. Put them in the front of your journal so you won't have to flip through everything to find all the good stuff. Start at your numbered pages and make the following templates and checklists:

1. Divide your page into three even rows with the "Why Is That?" Exercise at the top.

   Directly under that write the word *Challenge.*

   Directly under that write, "Why is that?"

   Just below the first line write, "Why?"

   Just below the second line write, "Why?"

2. At the top write, "Five questions to uncover your deeper magical need."

   Under that write following four questions:

1. Does this issue affect your financial well-being, your stability, or a physical item? (Prosperity)

2. Does this need make you feel vulnerable or at risk in any way? (Protection)

3. Is this need influenced or affected by another person or group of people? (Love)

4. Does this issue send you into anxiety just thinking about it? Does it trigger fear or inner resistance? (Healing). Are you looking to create a new path or avoid a block that was put in your path? Is there an obstacle that you keep running into? (Clearing)

3. At the top write, "Clarified Intent."

Under that write the following questions:

Why do you want that?

- Whose voice do you hear in your head when you think about that spell? Maybe it's your mother's voice or your teacher's voice.

- Does it come from your higher/divine self or from your ego?

- Do you understand why you want that?

- What does fulfillment look like?

What motivates this clarified want?

- How do you want to feel when this want is fulfilled?

- What does that feeling mean to you?

- What does that feeling validate or heal?

- Why do you need that healing or validation?

4. At the top write, "Words of Power Checklist."

Under that write the following bullet points:

- Intent

- Final Why

- Deeper Need

- Branch of Magic

- Deficit

- Keywords

- Story

5. At the top write, "Creating a Belief."

   Under that write the following bullet points:

   - Past tense

   - Signs of success

   - Statement of gratitude

   - Length of time before results

   - Signs of success

   Drop down a few lines and write, "Incantation."

   Under that write the following bullet points:

   - Two lines for what I am manifesting

   - Two lines for calling on assistance

   - Two lines for clearing out limits

   - Two lines for reaffirming what I am manifesting and closing the spell

   Drop down a few lines and write, "Affirmation."

   Under that write the following bullet points:

   - Past tense

   - Positive

- Leave an opening for growth

6. At the top write, "Candle Spell."

Under that write the following bullet points:

- Intent
- Candle type
- Size
- Color
- Moon phase
- Moon sign
- Prosperity Deficit

  Herbs/oils

  Crystal

  Tarot Card

- Protection Deficit

  Herbs/oils

  Crystal

  Tarot Card

- Love Deficit

  Herbs/oils

  Crystal

  Tarot Card

- Clearing Deficit

  Herbs/oils

  Crystal

  Tarot Card

- Healing Deficit

  Herbs/oils

  Crystal

  Tarot Card

  Accessories and actions

7. At the top write, "Guidance."

   Under that write the following bullet points:

   - Divination type

   - Questions asked—results—interpretation

   - Conclusion

   - Changes to make to spell

8. At the top write, "Candle Spell Observations."

   Under that write the following bullet points:

   - Flame

   - Candle burn

   - Candle drips

   - Smoke

   - Burn speed

   - Other observations

   - Disposal

9. At the top write, "Candle Spell Results."

   Under that write the following bullet points:

   - Daily observations and signs of success

   - Emotions and personal reactions

   - Daily gratitude

- Reactions from others

- What manifested

- Other observations

You take it from here. Record all the steps to creating your candle spell, what you are learning about yourself, your deeper needs, your spell, and the ingredients. Include your petition paper, candle labels, pictures of how it looked.

Maybe paper is not your thing. If so, start an electronic journal. You can even do this in a mobile app on your phone. Whatever you use, your future self will thank you.

THE INDEX OF
INSPIRATION

When the world is filled with unlimited options, we need a starting point to measure all of our choices from. The sample spells, potential ingredients, and spell accessories in this index are best used as triggers to your magic. They will inspire other thoughts and ideas of how your spell can work for you.

Open up the index at random pages and see what message you get and what magical vibration wants to be part of your spell for a little bibliomancy. Enjoy the ride, because magic should be fun.

SAMPLE CANDLE SPELL INDEX

Before you cast your candle spell, cleanse your space, set up your altar, call in your divine allies and any other spirits that will be helpful, and prepare yourself in body, mind, and spirit. All the candle magic examples assume you have done all of this before casting the spell. If the spell does not specify an oil, choose one from the list of herbs or go with a standard carrier oil like olive.

PROSPERITY, MONEY, AND MATERIAL-NEED SPELLS

May the Odds Be in My Favor—Winning a Prize Spell

Leave the Mega Millions lottery to the gods and chaos, and bring your focus to spells that are within your spheres of influence. This spell is effective for the smaller, local win—something like getting a grant, winning a 50/50 chance, or even coming out ahead at the local casino.

Candle Color: Yellow or orange for success and luck

Candle Type: Seven-day candle, blessed pillar, or seven votives to bring in the power of lucky 7

Dressing Herbs: Chamomile, parsley, five finger grass, pennyroyal, and savory

Dressing Oil: Olive oil and lemongrass

Accessories: Mercury dime, pair of dice, and small red flannel bag

Alternative Preblessed Candle: Motor City HooDoo Lucky 7

Instructions:

1. Do your setup before casting your spell.
2. On your altar, prepare your candle by drawing or scribing 777 on the side. Then turn the candle to the opposite side and scribe your name, what you want to win, and when you want it.
3. Blend the seven dressing ingredients together. You will need about two tablespoons total. As you are blending, say out loud what you want to win and when you expect it. State out loud what your life will be like after you win. Look at and talk about the success of this spell in past tense.
4. Rub half of the herb and oil blend on your candle(s), or sprinkle it sparingly on top of the seven-day candle. Rub some of the blend on the Mercury dime and pair of dice. Set the dice in front of your candle with a 5 and 2 showing on top and all sides adding up to a 7.
5. Place some of your herb mixture in the red flannel bag with the Mercury dime while stating your goal for this spell.
6. Light the candle while stating your goal for this spell. Run the red flannel bag over the heat of the flame, close it up, and place it next to your candle.
7. When you have to leave, extinguish the candle and carry the bag and dice with you. When you return, relight the candle and

place the bag and dice next to it. Burn the candle every day until it is consumed or you have achieved your goal.

Lucky Cat Spell

Black cats are the messengers of the gods and can be considered very lucky. Let go of past superstitions as they were created to make people afraid of magic and women dominating the beer market.

Candle Color: Black
Candle Type: Cat figure candle
Dressing: Fast luck oil; ginger, sassafras, and cinnamon (You can make the oil by placing the herbs in olive oil to infuse it for three days around the full moon.)
Accessories: none

Instructions:
1. Scribe your name and what you need luck for onto the candle.
2. Anoint the candle with fast luck oil.
3. Visualize your life after you achieve your goal and give thanks for your success.
4. Light the candle.

Hunting Money Spell

Hunting money is when you spend cash that has been anointed and charged up to return to you with friends. How cool is that? The more bespelled money you spend, the more it hunts up for you to put into your pocket. This is very useful for business owners as they buy supplies that will bring a large return.

Candle Color: Green, gold, or orange for money
Candle Type: Blessed money draw candle or any type of candle that is available
Dressing Herbs or Oils: Sage, cinnamon, date, sandalwood, and patchouli

Accessories: Spending money

Instructions:
1. Blend the herbs and oils. You will need about two tablespoons. You can use whatever combination of herbs and oils you have. If you do not have any of the oils, put the herbs in an olive oil or a cooking oil that is handy.
2. Place the money on your altar and sprinkle half of the blend on your money and anoint your candle with the other half. If you are using a blessed candle you can forgo this step.
3. Place your candle in its holder on top of the money and herbs. Light your candle and talk out loud about what you want your money to hunt.
4. Spend the money as you need to. You can add money that you want to bless to your pile as long as your candle is still burning.

Bills, Bills, Bills—Clearing My Debt Spell

If you cast this spell, you must spend what you plan on your intended target or the money will dry up. This is best done on a new moon, but you can start it whenever you need it as you will also be drawing and clearing.

Candle Color: White
Candle Type: Seven-day or any container candle. Can also use a blessed spiritual cleansing candle.
Dressing Herbs or Oils: Sage, sassafras, bay, cinnamon, and sandalwood
Accessories: List of bills or the actual bills, paper drawn as an oversized check

Instructions:
1. List your bills due in the next thirty days or collect them in a pile. Add them up and put that amount on the check you've created. Make the check from the universal bank of

abundance. Date the check for thirty days from now.
2. Blend your herbs and oils and sprinkle some onto your bills and the check you created. You can use whatever combination of herbs and oils you have. If you do not have any of the oils, put the herbs in an olive oil or a cooking oil that is handy.
3. Dress your candle with the herb blend and light the candle stating the amount you need and when you need it. Then say, "That or something better."
4. Place the last bit of your herbal blend into your wallet and the shoes you wear to work.

Daddy Warbucks—Business Success

Business success is more than luck. You are making decisions, creating value, and getting the cooperation of customers, staff, and investors. It is a symphony of energy that drives your success. This candle spell charges and blesses a charm to hang above your door and power that energy.

Candle Color: Yellow, blue, or gold
Candle Type: Pyramid, seven-day, or pillar candle
Dressing Herbs/Oils: Date, mustard seed, allspice, ginger, and jasmine

Accessories: Shredded money, poker chip, business card, citrine, red flannel bag, and pie tin

Instructions:
1. Blend herbs and oils with a pile of the shredded money. You can use whatever combination of herbs and oils you have. If you do not have any of the oils, put the herbs in an olive oil or a cooking oil that is handy.
2. Put a layer of shredded money in the pie tin. Scribe or draw on the candle the name of your business and the yearly, monthly, weekly, and daily revenue you are manifesting. Dress your candle with the herb blend and light the candle.
3. Put the herbal blend, poker chip, business card, and citrine in the red flannel bag. Run the bag through the flame and put it in front of the candle.
4. State your intent out loud. It is even better if you write a rhyming spell and say it nine times. Place your written intent or spell into the red flannel bag,
5. Let the candle burn as long as possible, relighting it every day. When the candle is consumed, place the bag above your most used outside door. Refresh this spell every quarter.

PROTECTION SPELLS

Rumor Has It—Stop Gossip Spells

Gossip saps your energy, and every time it is repeated you can feel the negativity created like an attack on your mind and spirit. This spell will take your name out of other people's mouths and make them forget all about what they wanted to say about you.

Candle Color: Black

Candle Type: Human figure candle, blessed protection candle, or any other black seven-day or pillar
Dressing Herbs/Oils: Hyssop, rosemary, fennel, nettle, rose
Accessories: none

Instructions:
1. Dress your candle with an herb/oil combination. You can use whatever combination of

herbs and oils you have. If you do not have any of the oils, put the herbs in an olive oil or a cooking oil that is handy.
2. State your intent or blessing out loud.
3. Light your candle and ask your guardians and protectors to take your name out of the mouths of people who wish you ill.
4. Extinguish your candle when you leave and relight it when you return.

Night Terrors Spell

Nightmares are draining. Whether they're from a stressful dream or a bad spirit feeding from you, night terrors can affect your health, mood, and clarity. This candle spell is to be done before bed and the candle extinguished before you settle down to sleep.

Candle Color: White or black
Candle Type: Blessed protection candle or devil figure candle, and a chime candle or tealight
Dressing Herbs/Oils: Frankincense, myrrh, eucalyptus, mint, and sandalwood
Accessories: Obsidian or other dark stone, scissors, holy water or Florida Water, plate or pie tin

Instructions:
1. Cleanse the scissors with the holy water or Florida Water.
2. Dress both the large and small candles.
3. Place the remaining herbs and the obsidian stone on the plate. Place the candles on top of the herbs and light them.
4. Open the scissors and run them through the flame of the candle. Place the scissors under the head of your bed, making sure they are open and pointing toward the top.
5. Call upon your guardians to clear your room and house of any harmful, negative energy and to create a barrier so none can come in.

6. Visualize your space filled with white light that creates a firm protective barrier. If you can, wait to go to sleep until the small candle is consumed. Extinguish any candle before you prepare for sleep. Set up a new chime or tealight every night to refresh the spell.

Fiery Wall of Protection Spell

When you are feeling particularly vulnerable, this spell not only burns away what has already been thrown at you; it also protects you from any other harm.

Candle Color: Red or orange
Candle Type: Any
Dressing Herbs/Oils: Ginger, peppermint, black pepper, geranium, juniper
Accessories: Cauldron or metal bowl and chalk

Instructions:
1. Scribe your candle with an equal-sided cross on four sides of the candle and then dress it with the herb and oil mixture.
2. Draw the same cross on the inside and outside of your cauldron or bowl on four sides. Place the herb and oil mixture in the bottom of the cauldron and the candle, too, lining up the crosses scribed on the candle and in the cauldron.
3. Place your cauldron in the room so that the crosses on the candle each face a wall, and use the chalk to draw a cross on the wall. Draw a cross on the opposite side of the wall and facing wall, cascading it through each room until you are placing a cross on the inside of an external wall. If you can, draw a cross on the ground directly below where the internal cross is.
4. Light the candle and visualize the fiery wall of protection activating each cross of protection all the way to the outside walls of where you live or work.

5. Let the candle burn as long as you can. When you need to extinguish it, state the following, "As I extinguish your flame in this realm, I light it in the spiritual to keep my protection strong and impenetrable." Relight your candle when you are able to attend to it. Once your candle is completely burned out, sprinkle any remaining herbs across your threshold, and use any remaining wax to draw a line across the threshold.

Blocking an Attack Spell

You will need two to four cups of dry sand, a small blessed and dressed protection candle of your choice, a piece of tissue paper with your name on it, a large box or baking sheet, a metal bowl, and a smaller box for disposal.

Place the large box or baking sheet on the floor and pour the sand into it. Place the paper with your name on it on top of the sand. Grind the paper into the sand until it becomes small shreds. While you do this, visualize cutting the connection to all people who wish you harm or to interfere with you. Use as much emotion as you can. They no longer influence your life.

Now scoop up the sand and paper mixture and put it in the metal bowl. Put a protection candle in the center. Say a prayer of protection or the blessing on the label. Light the candle and let it burn down to the sand and sputter out. (Never leave this candle unattended.) Transfer the sand to the smaller box and take to a dumpster far away from your home. Do this as soon as the candle sputters out. *Do not wait*. If you absolutely have to wait, then place everything in a plastic bag and seal it, disposing of it as soon as you can.

Protection from All Directions

You will need a blessed and dressed protection candle of your choice and a candle for each direction, five candleholders, your name on a clean sheet of paper, and sea salt (not table salt).

Create a circle of salt in the center of your altar—or use a big round pizza baking sheet to hold everything. Place the candleholders on the four directions of east, south, west, and north on the salt line and place a holder for the protection candle in the center.

Put the paper with your name under the protection candleholder. Put the protection candle in its holder and light it. Take the candle for the east and light it from the protection candle and place it in its holder.

Draw a line of salt from the east to all the other direction points—east to south, east to west, then east to north—while saying, "In all directions I am protected; from all sides I am protected. No words or thoughts can harm me."

Take the candle for the south and light it from the protection candle, touch it to the east candle, then place it in its holder. Draw a line of salt from the south point to the west point, then from the south point to the north point, then from the south point to the east point while saying, "In all directions I am protected; from all sides I am protected. No wishes or anger can harm me."

Take the candle for the west and light it from the protection candle, touch it to the east candle and the south candle, then place it in its holder. Draw a line of salt from the west to the north, then from the west to the east, then from the west to the south while saying, "In all directions I am protected; from all sides I am protected. No emotions or jealousy can harm me."

Take the candle for the north and light it from the protection candle, touch it to the east candle, the south candle, and the west candle, then place it in its holder. Draw a line of salt from the north to the east, then from the north to the south, then from the north to the west while saying, "In all directions I am protected;

from all sides I am protected. No actions or earthly forces or magic can harm me."

"As above, so below; as within, so without; I am protected, I am loved, and I am safe."

Sit with this spell for a while and feel yourself surrounded with protection, having built a fortress. When you are finished for the day, extinguish the candles and say, "I may extinguish your flame, but your magic glows brighter than the morning star."

Light these candles every day. The candle that burns the fastest is the direction from which your attack is coming. If you need further clarification, put a name on a paper next to each candle on the outside of the salt circle before you begin the ritual. The fastest-burning candle will tell you who the culprit is.

If the center candle burns the fastest, then it is someone very close to you, or you are sabotaging yourself.

Important candle-burning safety tips: Always remove all packaging around any candles before lighting them, and never leave a burning candle unattended. Do not leave a candle burning while you sleep. Blow it out and light it again the next day when you will be home to attend to it.

LOVE AND RELATIONSHIP SPELLS

New Love Spell

New love spells are a lovely open-ended opportunity to create your romantic wish list and have it met.

Candle Color: Pink, red, or green
Candle Type: Two blessed love candles, seven-day candles, or a series of votives
Dressing Oils: Lavender, clove, jasmine, peony, aloe
Accessories: Paper and pen, rose quartz stone

Instructions:
1. Write out your romantic wish list for a new love, including how you want to feel about them and when you are with them. Anoint that paper with lavender, and place it to the far right of your altar.
2. Write out a list of your own attributes, values, and how you like to make your partner feel. Anoint that with lavender. Place this to the far left of your altar.
3. Blend the clove, jasmine, peony, and aloe oils and dress one candle for the new love you are attracting and scribe "New Love for (your name)." Place the candle on top of the list that described your intended.
4. Use the oil blends and dress the other candle for you and scribe your name on it. Place the candle on top of the list that describes you.
5. Place the rose quartz in the center of your altar between the candles.
6. Light both candles and talk to them. Tell them what you're looking for in a partner and what you offer to a partner. Move the candles closer together and let the candles burn for at least three hours. (Make sure you can attend to them.)
7. The next day, light them again, and talk to them again about you and your new partner and how compatible you are together. Move the candles closer together and let them burn for at least three hours.
8. On the third day, light them again. Talk to them about how your values and personalities complement each other and how you are ready for the new love in your life. Move the candles so they touch the rose quartz.

Let the candles burn for at least three hours. Relight the candles every day until they are consumed.

Call Me Maybe—Come to Me Spell

A come to me spell has a specific person in mind when you are casting it. You are sending the message that you are definitely interested and ready for their attention. Come to me will draw them to you, but it can't make them love you. This is all about the initial pheromones that draw someone to you. It's up to you to land that fish by getting to know them, connecting where you are compatible, and encouraging love to grow.

Candle Color: Pink or blue
Candle Type: Seven-knob figure candle, blessed attraction candle, seven-day pink candle, or seven pink votives
Dressing Herbs: Catnip, damiana, orange blossom, patchouli, peony
Accessories: Seven pins, picture of your love interest, picture of yourself, rose petals, plate, and white or pink ribbon

Instructions:
1. Blend herbs with enough olive oil to make them stick to the candle. Dress your seven-knob candle and scribe your name on one side and your love interest's name on the other side. Place a pin in every knob of the candles.
2. Place rose petals on the plate and put the candle in the center with the name of your love interest to the left.
3. Put the picture of your love interest to the left of the plate and your picture to the right.
4. Light the candle and talk to it as if it is your love interest. Invite them to contact you. Tell them how interesting they are and how compatible you are. When a pin drops, you know

they have thought of you. Burn the candle until that knob is consumed.
5. Repeat this for six more days. On the seventh day, place the rose petals between your pictures, making sure they face each other. Roll up the pictures together, tie them with the ribbon, and seal with the last of the wax. Keep the picture on your altar until they call.

Get Lucky—Hot Date Spell (When You Are Single)

Whether you are in a relationship or not, sometimes all you want is a hot night (or day) of play, lust, passion, and fun. This hot date spell is all about your level of comfort being in play and it being matched by the other person(s).

Candle Color: Red or purple
Candle Type: Five votives
Dressing Herbs/Oils: Damiana, rose, nightshade, cinnamon, savory
Accessories: Candleholder, rose petals

Instructions:
1. Blend your herbs and oils. (You can blend the herbs in an olive or vegetable carrier if needed.) Tomatoes, potatoes, and peppers are all nightshades and perfectly acceptable for this spell.
2. Dress all five votives as you call in the energies of play, confidence, laughter, lust, and passion. Light one and put it in your bedroom to burn.
3. Take a bath in rose petals and feel how your confidence and sex appeal grow. (If you can't take a bath, create a spray bottle with warm water and rose petals and spritz your entire body.)
4. Let one votive candle burn until it is consumed. Repeat this process for five days or until your hot date happens—whichever comes first.

Sexy Times Date Night (When You Are in a Relationship)

Life gets busy, time passes, and you start to feel disconnected sexually from your partner. This quick spell may be just what Eros ordered.

Candle Color: Red
Candle Type: Votive (easiest is a blessed votive)
Dressing Herbs: Patchouli and peppercorn
Accessories: Apple

Instructions:
1. Core out a space in the apple for the votive candle.
2. If this is a plain votive, rub the votive with olive or vegetable oil and then dress it with patchouli and peppercorn and place it in the apple.
3. Call Aphrodite, asking for her help to heat up the lust between you and your partner.
4. Light the candle, clear your schedule, and make plans with your sweetie for the evening.

Awaken the Love Within

When you are feeling unloved and unlovable it's time to awaken the love within and reconnect with the divine energies of the universe. Once that love is awakened, you are a natural draw to more love and affection.

Candle Color: Orange
Candle Type: Blessed heart chakra candle, orange pillar, orange container candle, or four orange votives
Dressing: Sandalwood oil
Accessories: Heart symbols, image of lock with key (or actual lock and key)

Instructions:
1. Dress and set up your candle in its holder on your altar with the image of a heart in front of it.

2. Light the candle while saying, "Sacral chakra, glow and grow into a brilliant orange sphere filling me with divine love from the tips of my toes to the top of my head."
3. Hold on to the lock and key image and focus on the lock being your sacral chakra. Imagine a key fitting into the lock and unlocking it, releasing all the love that has been contained within you.
4. Repeat this daily until the candle is consumed.

Friends and Family

That's What Friends Are For—Be/Find a Good Friend Spell

Candle Color: Any color that represents friendship to you
Candle Type: One votive and three chime candles
Dressing Oils: Tangerine, basil, and vanilla
Accessories: Orange cut in half, bowl, three goblets, 3 of Cups tarot card

Instructions:
1. Juice the orange, keeping the skin of the half intact. Divide the juice between the three goblets.
2. Dress the candles and the half orange skin with the oil blend.
3. Place the orange in the bowl. Put the votive in the center of the orange and secure the chime candles around it. Place the tarot card in front of the bowl.
4. Light the candles and make three toasts with the goblets, drinking the juice as you go: The first is for friends past and the love and growth they brought to you. The second is for friends you have today, known and unknown. May you recognize the blessings they bring into your life and give blessings back to them. The third is for future friends. May you recognize them as they enter your

life. May you be a good friend and grow your friendships in return.

5. Let the candles burn and pool into the orange. Relight them every time you return home, toasting to friendship.

Marriage/Committed Relationship
Adam and Eve—Happy Marriage Spell

Love is a verb and long-lasting marriages know and act on this. This spell will fill your relationship with vibrations of happiness, commitment, and protect you from interference from others.

Candle Color: Purple or pink
Candle Type: Figure candles, blessed pillar or seven-day candle
Dressing Herbs: Comfrey, basil, and marjoram
Accessories: Honey, two cinnamon sticks, three figs, a plate, two rose quartz stones, happy picture of the couple

Instructions:
1. Blend your herbs with olive or vegetable oil. Dress your candles and place them on the plate.
2. Drizzle honey on the plate to remind you of the sweetness of life when you are working together.
3. Place the three figs (or dates) on the plate to ensure that you will never grow hungry.
4. Place the cinnamon sticks on the plate to transform any stress into support for each other.
5. Place the picture on your altar in front of the plate with the rose quartz on the picture.
6. Light the candles and give thanks for a loving relationship. If you are having trouble feeling it, state everything you are grateful for in your partner.

Faithful Partnership

This spell clears away the interference of others and brings the energy of love and cooperation into your marriage.

Candle Color: White
Candle Type: Seven-day
Dressing Herbs: Cumin, marjoram, and mint
Dressing Oil: Lavender
Accessories: Candleholder, red flannel bag, four-inch square of paper, happy picture of the couple

Instructions:
1. Blend the dressing herbs and oil and set half aside.
2. Dress your candle and secure the picture facing into the candle. Then place it in your candleholder.
3. Light the candle and say your words of power. Relight the candle every day until it is consumed.
4. Place a pinch of the herbs in the paper and fold it so it's self-sealing. Dip it in the molten wax. Put this packet in something your partner carries every day. Do it in a way they cannot easily find it. If this is not possible, sprinkle the herbs in their shoes.
5. Place the rest of the herbs in the red flannel bag and carry it with you. Invite your partner to contact you with loving words instead of spending that attention on someone else.

Truly, Madly, Deeply—Falling in Love Again Spell

It is so easy to let the busy-ness of life cloud the true feelings of love you and your partner have for each other. Couples drift apart, yet the unspoken love remains waiting for the invitation to fall back in love.

Candle Color: Red or purple

Candle Type: Marriage figure candle or appropriate figure candles
Dressing Oils: Cinnamon and jasmine
Accessories: Plate, red ribbon

Instructions:
1. Dress the candle(s), and tie a red ribbon around the candle(s) to contain the energy between you.
2. Place them on the plate and light them. As you light them, chant four times, "Truly, madly, deeply, we fall in love again."
3. Let the candles burn and relight them every time you return home. Remember to be loving from this moment forward to empower your spell.

CLEARING SPELLS

Break That Spell/Curse

When someone throws a curse on you, they are expecting you to break it with aggression and slap back and protect against it. Bursting out of it from the inside will be a surprise they never see coming.

Candle Color: Light color to white
Candle Type: Three votives around a white figure candle appropriate to you
Dressing Oils: Frankincense, lemongrass, myrrh
Herbs: Cinnamon, nettles, lemongrass
Accessories: Salt, plate, mirrors, baking sheet

Instructions:
1. Dress all candles with frankincense, lemongrass, and myrrh.
2. Dig out the bottom of the figure candle and load with cinnamon, lemongrass, and nettles.
3. Sprinkle salt on the plate and place your candles with the figure candle in the center and the votives circling it. Make sure they all touch.
4. Put the plate on a baking sheet, and place as many mirrors as possible, reflective side toward the candles, around your spell to amplify the energy you are creating.
5. Call in your divine self, guardians, and spirit guides to help in this spell.
6. Light all candles and watch them reflect the power of your divine light back upon themselves. The votives will cause the figure candle to melt faster. When the figure candle has burned halfway down, take down the mirrors, and your energy will blast the curse out of your body, aura, and energy.
7. Watch as the candles melt and burn down. Take note of any shapes in the wax that spill onto the plate or baking sheet. Make sure you are attending the candles on the final burn to contain any herbs that may catch on fire.
8. When you are done, scrape all remains into a garbage bag and throw it into a dumpster not associated with your home or work.

Blockbuster

Create an energetic firecracker and blow that block out of the way.

Candle Color: Red
Candle Type: Blessed pillar, seven-day, or plain pillar and seven short-burn candles like chimes or tealights

Dressing Oils: Dragon's blood, ginger, lemon-grass

Accessories: Paper and pen, firecrackers, outdoor altar, cast-iron cauldron or a firepit

Instructions:

1. Dress your candles with the blend of oils.
2. Set the seven-day candle and one chime candle on your outdoor altar. Light both.
3. Write out everything that is blocking you. Cry, rage, and scream your frustration onto the paper as you put down everything that is bothering you. Dress the paper with the dragon's blood, ginger, and lemongrass blend of oils.
4. Fold the paper and wrap it around a strip of firecrackers and place it in your cauldron or another safe place to allow it to burn.
5. Light the firecrackers from the chime candle's flame and stand back. Watch as they blow and feel your energetic blocks burst. (It's OK if you light a long match from the candle and then use the for the firecracker. Safety is best!)
6. Burn any remaining paper. Put the chime candle back on the altar. Stay outside as long as the chime candle is burning. Bring your tall candle into the house and keep it lit for as long as possible.
7. Repeat this six more times on different days as needed. Use a new chime candle with the same tall candle each time. Consecutive days on a waning moon are best.

House Clear and Balance

Candle Color: White and seven chakra colors

Candle Type: Blessed candle, plain pillar, or seven-day, and votives or chime candles

Dressing Herbs/Oils: Sage, peppermint, rosemary, pine

Accessories: Sage bundle, two buckets of water, spray bottle, salt, candleholders

Instructions:

1. Blend some of the herbs and oils in any combination available to you. If needed, use olive oil to blend the dry herbs in. Dress and light the tall white candle. Place it in a candleholder in the heart center of your home (where you spend most of your time). This candle will not move during the spell.
2. Fill the spray bottle with warm water and a quarter cup of salt.
3. Fill the two clean buckets halfway with cool clear water. Drop in peppermint and rosemary (oil or herb). Place the buckets in the center of the room.
4. Spray the room with salt water. Light the sage bundle and smudge the room. Walk the buckets around the room and into the next going counterclockwise in the room and in your home.
5. Repeat this in every room in the house counterclockwise. When you are done, walk the buckets counterclockwise to the main door you use, outside, and all the way off of your property. Dump the water into the street in a way that it will not run back to your house.
6. Return to the tall white candle. Dress and light the seven candles of different colors. One by one, walk them clockwise through each room of the house. Return them to the tall pillar and place them around it. When you are done, thank the spirits of the house.

MOON SIGN INDEX

Your most powerful lunar time is when the moon is in the sign you were born under. This lunar return is when you reenergize your spirit, rebalance your emotions, and bring your self-perception back to an empowered place. This is your personal beginning of the month, and you can plot out your magic for the rest of your magical month as the moon moves through its phases and the twelve astrological signs over the next twenty-eight days.

Your emotions are the battery to your candle spell. How you feel about something will make or break your spell, and the sign that the moon is in influences your emotions. Approximately every 2.5 days the moon moves into a new sign, affecting what your emotional focus is and giving you another opportunity to fine-tune your candle spell. Check your lunar calendar for the sign the moon is in and make that energy work with your spell. If it's not a great time, wait a day and you will get a different vibe to use to break through emotional patterns and blocks that stop your magic.

MOON IN ARIES

Aries is the "I Am" sign. When the moon is in Aries, this is the perfect time for self-improvement, motivation, and spells that involve the will. Give your magic some focus on the self, individuality, and personal energy.

Prosperity: Will bring a strong sense of self-worth to spells that affect your career path and people noticing your worth.

Protection: Will bring strength of will to your protection spells.

Love: Brings a strong sense of self-esteem and helps you understand what you really want from your relationships and let go of ones that will never bring that.

Clearing: Helps you let go of things that no longer define you or bring you an energetic return.

Healing: Leverage this energy to push through the hard parts of healing that make you want to quit.

MOON IN TAURUS

Taurus is the "I Have" sign. When the moon is in Taurus, this is the perfect time for money spells anchored in your personal values. Any candle spells that involve growing or cultivating are empowered with this moon sign.

Prosperity: Will bring a boost of growth and stability to your prosperity spells and align them with your personal value system to make them easier to manifest.

Protection: Protection spells that need to be stable, grow over time, and be rooted in reality will be empowered.

Love: Will bring a practical, grounded energy to relationship spells. Also a very good time for fertility.

Clearing: Will bring a grounded energy that helps you let go of illusions that were clouding your judgment. Use Taurus energy to grow a new, practical belief that will push out irrational fears.

Healing: This energy will get you in touch with your body and what it needs to thrive. Good time to start a weight loss spell.

MOON IN GEMINI

Gemini is the "I Think" sign. When the moon is in Gemini, any spell that involves communication, creativity, legal matters like signing documents, becoming inspired, or expanding the mind will be more effective.

Prosperity: Use for prosperity spells that involve contracts and finding creative solutions to problems.

Protection: Use in legal protection spells and where you need to protect channels of communication.

Love: A good time for spells that heal family relationships and clear communication in any relationship.

Clearing: Use to clear any misunderstandings, creative blocks, and gaslighting.

Healing: A great time for healing spells that involve expanding your mind. Really good for spells to help your medical professional find solutions to your health issues.

MOON IN CANCER

Cancer is the "I Feel" sign. When the moon is in Cancer, it is a perfect time for spells that create tranquility and a healthy home and family life.

Prosperity: Use in spells to bring financial ease to your home.

Protection: Will charge up family protection spells.

Love: Use in peace and ease spells for your household.
Clearing: Use when clearing discord in your home.

Healing: Use in healing spells for clearing out family abuse. Also an excellent time for fertility, healthy pregnancy, and childbirth spells.

MOON IN LEO

Leo is the "I Will" sign. The moon in Leo is the perfect time for creativity, vision, and leadership spells. Candle spells for success, fame, gambling, and lust are perfect in this moon sign.

Prosperity: Will bring bright energy to prosperity spells that give you recognition. Do all candle spells that bring you fame in this moon sign.
Protection: Will bring a boost to protection spells that stop gossip and protect your reputation. Will power up spells that involve protection of children.
Love: Will bring a hot sexy vibe to any love spells.
Clearing: Use this moon sign to burn away self-doubt.
Healing: Will bring a willful energy to healing spells to break through limitations on your self-esteem.

MOON IN VIRGO

Virgo is the "I Analyze" sign. The moon in Virgo is the time of month for health and new job spells. Its energy is beneficial for any type of ritual spell.

Prosperity: Will bring a boost of energy for new job spells, including expanding your customer base.
Protection: Will help you close all the loopholes in your protection spells.
Love: Will help you get clear on what you want in a love relationship.
Clearing: Will clear the chaos and create order out of it.
Healing: Use very powerful healing vibes in this moon sign to connect to your body and analyze what it needs. Do pet healing spells in this moon sign.

MOON IN LIBRA

Libra is the "I Balance" sign. The moon in Libra is a good time to do candle spells that affect partnerships, whether legal, marriage, business, or coworkers. This is a good time for legal spells that involve contracts and revenge or protection spells.

Prosperity: Will bring clarity and balance to prosperity spells that involve partners.

Protection: Will bring clarity for any legal, money, and business protection spells and support revealing who is working as an enemy.

Love: Will bring balance and clarity to happy marriage spells and help uncover any infidelity.

Clearing: Will clear any lies of gaslighting so you can see the balanced truth.

Healing: Will bring balance to your energy so you can let go of inner sabotage.

MOON IN SCORPIO

Scorpio is the "I Transform" sign. The moon in Scorpio is best for transformational spells and spells that deal with taxes and credit. This is the time of the month when you can easily find what is hidden and secret.

Prosperity: Will power up spells to return your money to you, uncover hidden resources, or secure a loan.

Protection: Will bring you protection from tax troubles and dangerous situations.

Love: Brings very lusty energy to love spells and will support ending relationships.

Clearing: Helps to clear your vision to see hidden knowledge and wisdom.

Healing: Will push your healing energy to a transformational state. It is supportive of healing family legacies.

MOON IN SAGITTARIUS

Sagittarius is the "I Seek" sign. The moon in Sagittarius is best used in spells that revolve around learning or teaching philosophy, higher understandings, and bringing a deeper connection to your beliefs. This is a perfect time to connect with divinity.

Prosperity: Will bring a boost of energy for spells to gain students.

Protection: Will bring a higher understanding of why you need this protection spell and what you need to learn from it.

Love: Brings understanding about how your relationship works.

Clearing: Helpful in clearing confusion around what you believe.

Healing: Deepens your connection to the divine forces of the universe.

MOON IN CAPRICORN

Capricorn is the "I Utilize" sign. The moon in Capricorn is the perfect time to do spells around your position in the world. Spells to overcome obstacles and get favorable results from the governments are perfect for this moon phase.

Prosperity: Will bring prosperity and success in everything you do.
Protection: Will bring protection to your reputation and social standing.
Love: Brings sentimental energy. Also brings structure and foundations to a relationship.

Clearing: Use this sign to remove negative people and influences that are blocking your success.
Healing: Helps you get out of your emotions to see the facts. Gets you into a wise mind state.

MOON IN AQUARIUS

Aquarius is the "I Know" sign. The moon in Aquarius is good for spells that are very social. This time can be used to stop gossip and empower friendship and general acceptance spells. This is also a time to powerfully affect circumstances that are beyond your control and put them back in your control. When you want spells to happen quickly or with a bang, do them when the moon is in Aquarius.

Prosperity: Will bring speed to your prosperity spells and a cumulative effect.
Protection: Will help you step into control over the situation.
Love: Helps you think outside of the box to bring new energy to the relationship.
Clearing: Will bring a big banishing and help you let go of who is draining your energy.
Healing: Brings a freedom to let go of other people's opinions about you.

MOON IN PISCES

Pisces is the "I Believe" sign. The moon in Pisces is not the best time to do any spells, unless you are either casting a confusion spell or a clarity spell when things are confusing. Use the moon in Pisces for spells to avoid going to jail or to the hospital.

Prosperity: Be careful of what you wish for as your beliefs are manifesting, not what you really need.

Protection: Will enhance protection from outside forces, self-sabotage, and self-harm.
Love: Will bring confusion and codependency to a relationship.
Clearing: Will power up your clearing to get rid of everything that is ready to go and make way for a new beginning.
Healing: Will end the struggle by helping you let go and start over again.

COLOR INDEX

The emotional vibrations triggered by colors make them a powerful tool in your magic. If you don't have a colored candle, you can add the color to your spell in other ways—paper, paint, fabric, and any other craft material you can think of.

The placement of the color is another factor you can play with. One color for your altar, another color under the candle or wrapped around the holder. You can add colored glass or petition paper or choose a particular color of flower or even furniture you are working on.

AQUA/TEAL

Prosperity, Clearing, Healing

I am calling this blend of blue and green out as a magical color. During the 2020 pandemic I found myself unconsciously bringing it into every area of my life, so I investigated why. Blue transforms anger and stress and green brings stability, promotes growth, and brings hope. At Coventry, this is the color of our emotional balance candle. All these things pointed to aqua as a color of prosperity, hope, and, of course, emotional healing. Experiment with aqua and teal in your magic and see how the vibration changes.

Prosperity: Aqua's vibration brings a stable growth to your prosperity. You may find new resources, more intuition around your financial stability, and new opportunities.

Protection: This is an emotionally protective color. Include aqua in spells where you are preventing mental manipulation or gaslighting.

Love: Aqua's vibration will support reconciliation, happy marriage, and friendship spells.

Clearing: With its close association with water, the vibration of aqua will help wash away what you are clearing.

Healing: Aqua's vibration connects you to any sacred healing waters that will help wash away what is ailing you in body, mind, emotions, or spirit.

BLACK

Protection, Clearing, Healing

Black is not on the color wheel as it isn't considered a color. Ha! Magic knows it as a color, and spellcasters use it frequently. In advertising it is seen as elegant, attractive, sophisticated, and exclusive. It is also culturally tied to death, negativity, and a lack of sensation. It's seen as both a lack of color and a concentration of color, making this a mutable energy to use.

Dark matter, the black expanse between the stars, is a new discovery in our cosmos, and there is a universe of unanswered questions about it. This brings me back to the vibration of black in magic: it contains the unknown and unknowing. This is powerful energy to use in protection, clearing, and healing.

Prosperity: I don't use black in prosperity work unless I am trying to shed light on my hidden resources or hidden knowledge.

Protection: As I said above, this is my go-to color for protection, because I am unseen when I use black. If people don't know where to aim, how will they hit me? I also see black as an all-absorbing and transforming color that my inner sci-fi geek turns into a black hole that spits what was sent my way out into another galaxy. I'll let that attacker wear themselves out until they forget about me.

Love: This is an antilove color that creates a lack of sensation. Unless you are a stalker that wants to stay in the shadows, black is not a good choice here. (And don't be a stalker—nobody wants that.)

Clearing: Bring on the black when I am clearing. I use black to show me what needs clearing. I imagine fingerprint dust on the offending energy, and voilà, I grab on to it and push it out. I also use black as a protective shield when I am opening up to clearing.

Healing: Sometimes you need to step into the unknown when you are healing big issues. Use a black candle to represent sending light into the dark corners. You can also use black or grey to cool energy that needs a little shade to settle down in.

BLUE

Healing, Clearing

The vibration of blue will change depending on the hue. It is the color of calm, security, authority, and trust, but also depression. It is seen to be a very productive color; in its softer hues it is often used in offices. It is a transformative color as it can calm violent aggressive feelings as well as bring inspiration out of chaos. Darker blues are more mental, and the lighter blues are more lunar and emotional. Bright blue is also the color of the throat chakra, promoting communication and speaking your truth. Indigo blue is the color of the third-eye chakra, bringing understanding, visions, and psychic development.

Prosperity: Use blue in prosperity spells when you need to balance logic and intuition, require more inspiration, or have a legal component. This is also an authoritative color when establishing your team.

Protection: When you need protection in legal matters while pursuing spiritual development or while working on dream magic, blue is a good choice.

Love: In spells that bring tranquility and peace to the environment or relationship, light blue is an excellent choice.

Clearing: Blue soothes and cools emotions. It brings peace, calm, and harmony to clearing spells that have lots of emotional upset.

Healing: Spiritual development, dream work, and gaining wisdom all vibrate stronger with all shades of blue.

BROWN

Prosperity, Protection, Healing

The earthy vibrations of brown are very grounding, nurturing, and supportive. When thought of, brown is most likely to bring the feelings of reliability, resilience, dependability, strength, and security, making this an excellent color for spells that deal with the home, pets, court cases, and self-esteem issues.

Prosperity: When you need to bring stability to your prosperity, add a brown candle to your spell. This is very useful when it seems like the more money you bring in, the faster it goes out.

Protection: Stability is the vibration of brown. All protection work must have a stable foundation, and I have found that in certain cases, stability is all that is needed to shore up the protection magic.

Love: Brown won't incite passion, but it will help with bringing a groundedness to relationships of any kind. Family foundation issues and even friendship magic are helped by brown vibrations. Pet blessings and other spells are in the companionship category, and brown is the color that pets respond to energetically.

Clearing: Not a clearing color, brown will however send to earth what you are getting rid of so it doesn't have a chance to reattach to your energy.

Healing: Healing magic done with a brown candle will recruit the help of nature spirits and Mother Earth to bring balance to your energy. It creates a solid foundation to start your healing journey on.

GOLD

Prosperity, Healing

Chime candles often come in a gold dip. Gold is associated with the sun, male energies, and riches. If it's not metallic gold, refer to the magical associations of orange or yellow.

Prosperity: Wealth, riches, and royalty are all the vibration of gold. Use in money spells to bring fast luck.

Protection: Topping your protection spell with a gold candle brings success to your magic.

Love: Use gold in love spells to bring a dazzling energy—or if you are looking for a proposal.

Clearing: Gold will increase the speed of the clearing magic you are doing.

Healing: Gold brings balance to your healing spell. It calms difficult situations and gets everyone working in the same direction.

GREEN

Prosperity, Love, Healing

Green is a money color, and not because of the color of US paper currency, but because of the energy of growth and abundance that it vibrates with. Green stimulates growth, stability, and sustainability. Think about the green of spring, the lushness and abundance of summer, the deep green of the evergreen trees. Using a green candle for your spell brings the vibration of growth to ensure that you can harvest what you are working toward. Green is calming, motivating, natural, and optimistic. It is also the color of the heart chakra and can help transform your fears into strengths.

Prosperity: All prosperity candles I make are green; it is also my favorite color. I love the welcoming energy of green. It is universal, inclusive, and equalizing, making it a very powerful growth and abundance energy.

Protection: Green works with protection by gaining the blessing of nature and bringing a calm strength. Dark green brings the everlasting energy (think evergreens) to survive the onslaught of an attack.

Love: The heart chakra is green, making this an excellent choice for self-love and healing love spells.

Clearing: Green replaces more than it clears. It will push out what is not working for you and replace it with loving, abundant energy.

Healing: The emerald green of the heart chakra is transformative, making this a lovely color for healing work that addresses your fears and limitations. Green and healing also go together when dealing with prosperity and food issues.

ORANGE

Prosperity, Love, Healing

Red and yellow make an energetic orange (my second favorite color). The aggressive nature of red is tempered with the logic and communication of yellow, creating confidence that feeds luck, business spells, career spells, and overall success spells. Energy, enthusiasm, attention, happiness, personal power, compassion, and encouragement resonate with orange, making this a very adaptable color. It is also the color of the sacral chakra, which rules love and passion.

Prosperity: Use an orange candle in business and career spells, especially if they need a boost of speed to manifest. Use in spells where you need encouragement, a stronger will, courage, and the stamina to get the deed done.

Protection: Orange is not a protection color, as it attracts attention. If you add orange to your protection spells, do it sparingly and focus its energy on a successful spell. Still, I have been using orange in my travel spells because my luggage is orange and I find it has been successful in making sure I am well cared for, people see me on the road, and my luggage arrives safely.

Love: Orange is a love color as it has the attraction power of red and the smooth talker energy of yellow. This is a good choice for a hot date candle or a fall in love all over again spell. Its association with the second chakra makes orange a good choice for spells that call to a new love as well as healing your own intimacy fears.

Clearing: Orange is not a clearing color as it has too much attraction energy. Adding orange into a clearing spell will pull in energy, so make sure you have defined what energy will offset what is being cleared.

Healing: Use orange in healing spells that need vitality, courage, willpower, and passion. Healing love and self-esteem issues will benefit from an orange candle.

PINK

Love, Healing

The Women's March of 2017 owned the color pink and reclaimed it as a color of feminine empowerment. Previously relegated to romance or a young girl's fashion and toy choices, pink is now more respected and empowered for many uses. Pink has a naturally calming vibration that allows you to step into the joy of romance, kindness, creativity, and innocence. Thinking about it, the Women's March of 2017 is considered one of the most peaceful marches in history; maybe the vibration of pink helped that come to pass. If pink is your favorite color, use it as much as possible and let it power up every branch of your magic.

Prosperity: Not a color associated with prosperity. Incorporating pink into a prosperity spell will bring a calm, nurturing energy.

Protection: Using the color pink for protection may be counterintuitive, but after the power raised by millions of women on January 21, 2017, use pink to tap into that goddess protection power.

Love: Romance is the love vibration of pink. Pink's vibration brings a gentle, nurturing caress of love and romance, leaving the power of passion to red, orange, and at times purple. Every love spell benefits from pink, so experiment with the difference between pink and red in your love spells.

Clearing: If you choose a pink candle for a clearing spell, you will bring in calm energy that will gently let go of what needs to be cleared. If you are dealing with a highly emotionally charged issue, starting with pink for a first pass at clearing will help get all parts of the self—body, mind, emotions, and spirit—in agreement for the clearing.

Healing: Pink's vibration attracts a gentle angelic energy that is helpful in any healing spell. Pink's nurturing vibration encourages healing in highly emotionally charged situations.

PURPLE

Prosperity, Clearing, Healing

If you want to do something in a big way, purple's vibration expands anything you desire. One of the ways purple does this is by clearing from you the limitations your fears and blocks may have put on your success. The logic of blue blends with the action of red, creating motivation and bravery to accomplish your goals. Purple is the color of wealth and royalty, helping you fully step into your innate magical power. Purple is also the color of the crown chakra, bringing in divinity and wisdom.

Prosperity: When you need to step into your own authority and expand upon your original goal, purple's vibration supports that.

Protection: The vibration of royalty brings protectors. Use purple to secure the support and protection of the people around you.

Love: Lighter shades of purple can be successful with love magic. For fidelity and happy marriage spells, it brings a purity of intent and loyalty from all parties.

Clearing: Purple's vibration naturally pushes out impurities and inner sabotage to replace it with a divine blessing.

Healing: There is a spiritual peace brought forth with the vibration of purple. It promotes healing in every level by invoking divine connection and blessing.

RED

Love, Prosperity, Healing

Red is the most visible color due to its long wavelength. You notice it before you notice any other color, making it perfect for warning signs that need your immediate attention. It is also the most energetic color and can incite an immediate emotional reaction. The attention it draws and the energy it emits make it magnetic to attract what you want. In contrast, it can also heat up and drive away energy when directed to. Red is also the color of the root chakra, bringing empowered grounded energy to everything you are striving for.

Prosperity: Use red in prosperity spells to magnetize your intention and draw it to you. It also brings the stamina for a particularly difficult project. You can also apply red to create a burst of energy to break through a block. Red energy can speed up your prosperity spells.

Protection: In protection spells it warns others that to approach is dangerous to them. Red is the color of anger, war, and battles. It sends up the flare that you are not to be trifled with as it is the color of courage and victory.

Love: Passion, heat, sexuality, fertility, and aggressive feelings all come with the color red. Using this in love spells will cause them to burn hot and fast.

Clearing: Choose red when you need to burn something away or aggressively cut and clear it from your life.

Healing: Red is aligned with the element of fire, and it brings vitality, vigor, and intense health.

SILVER

Healing, Clearing, Protection

Metallic silver is often used to represent divine light and the balance it brings to your energy. Silver has a very lunar vibration and connects you to the continual ebb and flow of life. If the candle is not metallic, it will vibrate the neutral color of grey.

Prosperity: Silver may not represent wealth, but it does bring in a vibration of balance in all efforts to ensure a return on investment at a future date.

Protection: Silver repels negativity and reflects it back to its source.

Love: The silver anniversary represents twenty-five years of marriage. Silver brings patience and perseverance to love spells.

Clearing: The vibration of silver is naturally clearing. It will pull out energy that is harmful and repel additional negative energy.

Healing: Silver has been used, in times past, to prevent infections, which tells us that it has an innate healing vibration. Use silver to bring in a vibration that will clear you of disease and rebalance your aura and vital energy to a healthy state.

WHITE

Healing, Protection, Clearing, All-Purpose

White has been traditionally used as an all-purpose candle. If you can't find the color you want, go to white. That is because it is seen as a clear slate, sterile, empty, or innocent of any specific vibration. It is also seen as the color of purity—to bathe yourself in white light is to bring divine blessings. Because of its purity, this color is excellent in cleansing spells.

Prosperity: White in prosperity spells represents a clean slate, starting anew, or being a vessel for the spell you are creating.

Protection: Representing surrounding yourself with divine protection, white is a popular color for protection spells.

Love: White in love spells represents pure love. Use in spells to clear past hurts and start over with your loved one.

Clearing: A favorite of mine for clearing. It will act like a magnet to draw out what needs to be cleared and refill you with divine protection.

Healing: White light for healing work brings in a purity and can also leave you a little cold and clinical. This all-purpose color needs direction when you are doing healing work and takes that direction very well.

YELLOW

Prosperity, Healing

Yellow is a high-energy color that can speed you to success or irritate the crap out of you. Its extroverted warmth brings mental clarity, communication, creativity, confidence, and courage.

When directed with your intent, yellow's vibration can power up your success spells and bring more notoriety in your career or community. It is associated with the air element, carrying the vibration of intellect and communication. It is the color of the solar plexus chakra where confidence, will, and personal power live.

Prosperity: Success, careers, and fame all benefit from the vibration of yellow. Use in spells where you need to be noticed above all others. This is also an excellent color for mental pursuits and when you need to be creative. Feel free to play with shades of yellow to find what works best for you.

Protection: Not a color for protection, yellow is more the hue for being a target as it gets you noticed. If you use yellow in a protection spell, make it the distraction that will pull the attacker's attention away from you.

Love: Use yellow in love spells where you want to get noticed and heat up the energy between you.

Clearing: Not a traditional color for clearing, but you can use yellow to harness the sun's energy to illuminate what is hiding from you and burn away attachments.

Healing: The vibration of yellow brings an abundance of energy to your healing spells. This is also a powerful color for communication; use it when you are healing your voice so you can speak your truth into the world. It is light, encouraging, and warm and helps you connect with the courage needed to complete your healing process.

MAGICAL HERB INDEX

Let me be clear: this is a *magical* herb index. At no time am I referring to any medicinal uses of the herbs—including ritual ingestion. Read this index with the mindset that you are creating a magical blend of herbs and oils that you will rub on, put around, and sprinkle on your candle. I chose the following small sampling herbs as they are, for the most part, easily attainable and may even already be in your kitchen. Magically using herbs can be straight out of the book, or it can be a journey of personally connecting with the ingredients to discover how they work with you. The descriptions in this guide are an amalgamation of what I have learned through reading and what I learned from the herbs. If you disagree with anything I have written, that is wonderful—it means you have your own unique relationship with that plant. Seriously, someone at some time in the past picked up that plant and decided what magic it is good for. That's all well and good, but you can also be the decider

in your own magic and feel your connection to the energy.

If you are inspired, dig deeper into the magical lore of herbs. There are some amazing books specifically on herbal magic that I often reference, and I will list them at the end of this index.

As you are reading, you will see many references to protecting from evil and cleansing evil, exorcism, hexes, curses, and such. Do I believe there is that much hexing in the world? Maybe? I first look at these evil energies as things that may be surrounding you that are discordant or disruptive to your vibration or the vibration of the spell you are casting. I also look at curses and negative energy as a sign that you have beliefs that need upgrading as they are connecting to energy that limits you. I look for energy that you may have crossed yourself up with, such as inadvertently picking up something nasty in your last adventure, and only lastly do I look for negative energy that may have been thrown at you.

AGRIMONY

Protection, Clearing

An excellent antihexing herb, agrimony clears energy from any negative intentions including your own. It helps relieve the stress caused in dramatic emotional situations and brings your emotions into balance.

Prosperity: Counters negative energy that affects your money including jealousy, envy, and your own insecurities.

Protection: This is the superpower of agrimony: clearing out and protecting you from all forms of negative energy. Use this in your protection when you are doing any spell or healing work.

Love: When your relationships are stressed, agrimony can help clear destructive energies such as anger, jealousy, envy, or obsession.

Clearing: Let go and let agrimony clear your inner and outer vision so you can see the truth of things to help you release the obsessive, anxiety-ridden negative energy around you. It will help clear entities and spirits, reverse spells, and break hexes.

Healing: To keep you from absorbing your client's energy, use the oil of agrimony on your hands. In your healing spells, agrimony can alleviate emotional discomfort, easing inner voices and thoughts. For dreaming and sleep spells, agrimony will help relieve stress and anxiety created in the mind and preventing sleep.

ALLSPICE

Prosperity, Love, Healing

Allspice is all about building confidence, reenergizing, stimulating, and charging up your magic. This is in my top five ingredients in money magic and love magic. *Go for it!*

Prosperity: Excellent money and luck herb because it will help to increase your vital and magical energy. Allspice will open the door to the opportunity you are looking for and then reenergizes you and stimulates your determination so you can take advantage of it.

Protection: The determination and strength of allspice bring a deeper commitment to your protection spells.

Love: When your energy is refilled, your stress relieved, and self-confidence boosted, it is easier to see the love that already surrounds you and opens you up to more love.

Clearing: The contented and positive energy brought by allspice displaces anxiety and emotional blocks.

Healing: Energize your healing spells with allspice, which unwinds tension and fills the aura and spirit with the energy needed to heal.

ALOE

Healing, Clearing

To many, this is a plant sent to us by the gods, as it has so many practical uses in life and healing qualities and keeps you connected with the divine.

Prosperity: Aloe jumps right in and connects you to the laws of Universal Abundance. It's

presence in your life as a live plant brings luck.

Protection: Protection from the divine is powerful and hard to penetrate. Aloe provides this by connecting you to the divine within and will guard against evil influences.

Love: The divine connection that aloe brings is very soothing to those who are lonely and looking for connection with others.

Clearing: Bad luck is quickly cleared with aloe as it cannot stick to you. Allow aloe's slick quality to clear out old issues that keep you stuck in the past and cool tempers.

Healing: Cooling, soothing, patient energy comes from aloe, helping to heal in body, mind, and spirit.

ALTHEA ROOT (MARSHMALLOW)

Love, Clearing, Healing

This herb draws positive spirits that work to bring balance to your emotions. The inner strength and fortitude of althea root counter and clear the excessive grief that can stop you from seeing the divine and loving connections in your life.

Prosperity: Althea root will draw in helpful spirits and ease emotional distress that prevents you from seeing the opportunities and growth in your life. Use it to help you find prosperity in the midst of trauma.

Protection: Draw in the helpful spirits that will strengthen your protection spells. Althea root is particularly good when you are protecting your heart and your mind from manipulation and influence.

Love: When you are feeling heartbreak and grief, althea root will bring balance and clear confusion, while retaining a loving connection. It will help strengthen friendships, helping you see the healthy energetic connection.

Clearing: Use althea root in your spells and rituals as a purification herb for body, mind, and spirit. It clears grief and overwhelming emotions and will also help you see the true intentions of the people around you.

Healing: Healing overwhelming grief is one of the superpowers of althea root. Use it to help you block overstimulation and bring the inner strength needed to persevere through your troubles.

ANGELICA

Protection, Love, Healing

Angel is the keyword in angelica, connecting you to the angelic realm—specifically archangel Michael. It imparts a healthy, vibrant aura that radiates with joy and love and clears out fears.

Prosperity: If you want to be filled with an abundance of good energy, add angelica to your spell. It does this by clearing out fears, bringing an understanding of your value, and evoking angelic help. Carry it for luck and to see other paths to your goal.

Protection: Use in spells that call to the angelic realm and your guardian angels to fortify your protection in all directions and against all forms of evil. It's a critical ingredient for spells that protect children and pregnant women.

Love: The vibration of angelica helps you see your inner light and personal value as well as the value of others. Understanding this clarifies relationships and gives you the strength to get out of unhealthy and abusive situations.

Clearing: Curses and hexes cannot exist in the presence of the divine. Angelica invites angels into your space, displacing harmful intent, energy, and spirits.

Healing: Brings a positive outlook on life that supports all levels of healing. Angelica is very important when you are protecting, clearing, and healing victims in abuse situations.

ANISE

Protection, Love, Healing

This is in the top five of the psychic enhancement and development ingredients as it protects you as you grow in ability.

Prosperity: Anise of all types helps you clear out the feelings of not being deserving by bringing in divine blessings.

Protection: Use anise to protect your psychic centers from overloading. It is employed in spells to protect from the evil eye, nightmares, evil spirits, and overall negativity.

Love: Anise brings the blessings of a long marriage by easing tensions and replacing stress with loving vibrations and happiness. This is also a wonderful ingredient to help one find romance.

Clearing: The protective energy of anise makes it a natural addition to clearing work for any negative energy, spirits, or influence.

Healing: The psychic superpower of anise enhances your sense of connection with the universe, thus bringing happiness and self-love.

ARNICA

Prosperity, Healing

Arnica's vibration brings the balance needed for success to any situation. It will clear what is preventing balance and draw the energy needed to restore it.

Prosperity: Arnica ensures a successful outcome of your magic and keeps you focused on finishing all the long-term steps for its success. It will also protect your project or spell from sabotage and negative wishes.

Protection: The balancing energy of arnica prevents spirits from entering a space where their influence will be detrimental. It also strengthens your spirit to protect against psychic attacks and energy drains.

Love: Arnica creates a protective barrier around your relationship against energetic attacks and curses.

Clearing: It clears negative energy by bringing in a higher vibration.

Healing: Arnica's reputation for healing physical accidents proves its healing vibration that helps clear the trauma from the event. It connects you with your core inner power and strength.

BALSAM OF PERU (RESIN AND OIL)

Love, Healing

The resin of the balsam of Peru is warming to your heart center. It is calming and uplifting and helps you feel a deeper connection to your own spirit.

Prosperity: Use in prosperity spells to warm your spirit, bringing confidence and motivation to your spell.

Protection: Add confidence and stability to your protection spells and strengthen your aura with balsam of Peru.

Love: Use this resin in your love magic to bring in the warmth of love, inner peace, connec-tion, and the ability to see all the potential of any relationship, This resin will instill you with self-compassion to cut through the expectations and codependency that another may have hooked into you with.

Clearing: When you are in the place of con-fidence and peace that is vibrated with this resin, you can let go of the issues that are keeping you in a state of stress.

Healing: The spirit of balsam of Peru releases tension and stress, helping bring comfort and peace of mind.

BASIL

Prosperity, Love, Healing

I am in love with basil as it supports success in every branch of the Magic 5. It is a plant that is worth having in your home so you can fill it with the magic of basil.

Prosperity: The energy of basil opens the path to wealth by attracting customers and busi-ness opportunities and keeps the negativity at bay. This is an herb of luck.

Protection: The blessings of basil make it impos-sible for evil to reside where basil is. Use basil in personal protection spells.

Love: Basil brings in the energy of compassion and cooperation making this an excellent herb for marital bliss. The peace, love, and confidence of basil are perfect for love spells.

Clearing: Basil's magic replaces sorrow with hap-piness. It reduces mental fatigue and makes it easier to cut through a cluttered mind.

Healing: Use basil in spells for happiness and peace in the family. The powers of basil instill courage, confidence, strength, and balance, making it an excellent herb for all levels of healing.

BAY LEAVES

Prosperity, Protection, Clearing

Where would Caesar be without his crown of laurel (bay leaves)? Less victorious for sure! Do you need to power up? Grab your bay leaves.

Prosperity: Any financial and material gain spell needs a bit of bay for victory, empowerment, success, and wish fulfillment.

Protection: Bay's vibration of power dispels evil and wards off negativity.

Love: Bay is a symbol of familial love and comfort. Use in spells to find true love and to protect your family from the storms of life.

Clearing: Used in purification ceremonies, bay's energy will clear out extreme emotions.

Healing: To increase clairvoyance and bring clarity to psychic visions.

BERGAMOT

Prosperity, Healing

Don't have bergamot available? Grab some Earl Grey tea and find a moment of happiness.

Prosperity: Bergamot vibrates happiness that is a magnet for positivity. This magic seed of prosperity grows fast. Use it in money draw spells to ensure that all money spent returns multiplied.

Protection: Bergamot helps keep your stressors in perspective.

Love: Bergamot brings happiness to all love and cooperation spells to help relationships grow in a healthy way.

Clearing: When you pull in positive energy with bergamot, there is no room for doubt.

Healing: Bergamot uplifts the spirit, relieving depression and tension from everyday living.

BLESSED THISTLE

Protection, Clearing

This prickly herb is truly blessed. It brings protection for body, mind, spirit, and emotions.

Prosperity: When requested, blessed thistle can be motivating and bring creative inspiration.

Protection: The prickly nature of blessed thistle is very protective, aggressively so. It will break hexes and keep all negativity away.

Love: Use blessed thistle in spells to keep unwanted attention away.

Clearing: The energy-repelling nature of blessed thistle results in clearing oppressive energy that can cause confusion and depression.

Healing: As blessed thistle sends away baneful spirits, it makes room and calls to helpful spirits. You will find more energy and connection to your divine self.

CARDAMOM

Protection, Healing

Surprise, your spice drawer just became more helpful! Cardamom brings the energy of perseverance, passion, and clear thought.

Prosperity: Include cardamom in spells that need the passionate energy to complete a project and move through the difficulties.

Protection: Employ this vibration for overall protection, especially around relationships.

Love: Use cardamom to heat up lust and passion. Everyone gets amorous when cardamom is around.

Clearing: Flip the script and turn to cardamom to clear away the fears that keep you separated from your environment and passions.

Healing: The healthy heat of cardamom stimulates the body and mind, bringing clarity of thought.

CATNIP

Prosperity, Love, Healing

Catnip carries a chill vibration that helps you connect with your inner strength and power.

Prosperity: Use catnip in spells to bring confidence and luck.

Protection: The vibration of catnip is very protective of children.

Love: Catnip has an affinity to feminine energy: it will heat up a woman's appeal and be very charming to the one you want to attract. The chill vibe of catnip is also great in friendship spells.

Clearing: Catnip's energy clears the chaos that keeps everyone on edge.

Healing: Use catnip in spells to center yourself to help you understand and connect with your own personal power and influence.

CAYENNE, CHILI PEPPERS, AND PAPRIKA

Protection, Clearing

Cayenne, chili peppers, and paprika are all from the hot pepper family. They all have subtle differences in their energy, yet their core magical purpose is too similar to differentiate them.

Prosperity: Use in prosperity spells to heat up the other ingredients, speed up the process, and open the road to success.

Protection: All of these chilies are a powerful addition to your protection spells. They cleanse negativity, including breaking hexes, and set a protective barrier.

Love: This is some undiluted heat to power up your passion and love spells.

Clearing: The negativity these peppers clear will free you from self-doubt and the obstacles you put in your own path.

Healing: When you add one of these peppers to your spell, you feel your spiritual connection to all of life in a deeper way.

CEDAR

Prosperity, Protection

The deep roots of the cedar tree bring the energy of stability and spiritual strength. Its energy connects heaven to the earth, making all things possible.

Prosperity: Cedar brings the energy of abundance, mobility, fertility, and strength. This vibration brings blessing to help manifest dreams and wishes.

Protection: Cedar is very protective from outer and inner discord. The balanced energy it brings will stabilize your protection.

Love: Use cedar to bring balance to your love relationships and grant a few wishes in the area of love.

Clearing: Big cedar energy purifies the spirit and clears anxiety, irritation, anger, and fears. Use in spells to removes the influences of others and clear obsessive thoughts.

Healing: This divine wood is used in consecrating any magical tool. Its grounding energy brings the self into balance, aligning body, mind, and spirit.

CELERY SEED

Healing, Clearing

Strengthening the mind is the magical superpower of celery seed.

Prosperity: Add celery seed if you are afraid of making a decision. Its vibration will help clear your head so you can see the way forward.

Protection: Celery's vibration protects you from being overwhelmed by spiritual downloads of information.

Love: This strong mind vibration of celery seed helps you see the bigger picture and the truth of the relationships in your life.

Clearing: Cut the confusion of information overload with the energy of celery seed so you can get to the heart of the matter.

Healing: Celery seed's vibration helps increase your psychic intuition and enhances all of the clairs (clairvoyance, clairaudience, clairsentience, etc.).

CHAMOMILE

Prosperity, Clearing

Chamomile's magical and medicinal properties are at opposite ends of the spectrum. Instead of the calming you may be used to with chamomile tea, magically, chamomile is hot, lucky, and vibrant.

Prosperity: The gambling luck energy of chamomile draws money. The riskier the proposition, the better it works.

Protection: Use chamomile to break a money jinx, including one you may have put on yourself.

Love: Invite in the calming energy of chamomile to emotionally balance everyone during reactive arguments and long-standing fights.

Clearing: Chamomile's vibration clears away sabotage and strengthens protection.

Healing: Chamomile will energize all other healing herbs and ensures a healing environment.

CINNAMON

Prosperity, Love

Cinnamon is a top-five must for your magical herb cupboard. As you will see, it's useful in many spells.

Prosperity: Cinnamon's high vibration is very useful in all prosperity, money-drawing, and road-opening spells. It will relieve the stress and nervous exhaustion that money issues bring, which in turn block your prosperity.

Protection: Protection spells are powered up with the energy of cinnamon. It will protect the mind from unwanted influence.

Love: Cinnamon's aphrodisiacally magic power comes from clearing the stress, melancholy, and anxiety that destroy confidence and decrease sexual passion.

Clearing: Use the high vibration of cinnamon to clear the energy and emotions that keep you stuck in a lower vibration.

Healing: Cinnamon is used in anointing oils to raise spiritual vibrations to a higher level and draw divine blessings. This in turn naturally enhances your abilities for psychic communication.

CITRUS (LEMON, LIME, ORANGE, GRAPEFRUIT, TANGERINE)

Prosperity, Healing

Oranges, lemons, and all citrus are very magical and must be included here. Each type in this family has its own signature magic outside of the uplifting and cleansing magic that is in all citrus. Explore the differences in your magic.

Prosperity: Citrus energy brings luck, wealth, abundance, and joy. Use any citrus fruit, specifically the dried peel, in any money spell as it will clear away what is stopping your

success and fill you with the energy to complete the project.

Protection: The vibration of citrus brings protection through its ability to spiritually clear an area.

Love: Sweetness and joy energies abound in all citrus, making this an interesting addition to love spells. They can sweeten someone up to you, but lemon can be used sour a relationship.

Clearing: The clearing power of citrus is great. It pushes out any disharmony and intense negative emotions.

Healing: A clear mind, open heart, vital energy, lifted spirits, and unending joy are the core magic in all citrus fruit. Use citrus in a happy home spell, heart-healing spell, and anything where joy will help remedy the situation.

CLOVE

Prosperity, Love

Clove is another must-have in your magical kitchen. The energy of clove is very money drawing, confidence building, and luck inducing.

Prosperity: Like all spices, clove's vibration is very money drawing. It's through its calming, confidence-building energy that it makes all things possible.

Protection: Clove's diverse magic is protective of the home and guards the residents from gossip.

Love: Clove has an energy that promotes friendship and community through strengthening self-confidence in all. With its lucky vibration, spells to meet a new love interest may benefit from clove.

Clearing: The calming property of clove can be used to clear the fears that block your success and negative influence. Clove is often used in clearing and blessing a spiritual working space.

Healing: Clove lifts your mood and spirit, calms nerves, brings confidence, and lessens the emotional pain of a troubling situation.

COMFREY

Protection, Clearing, Healing

Much of the magic purpose can be found in the name of *comfrey*—"to comfort." From releasing old beliefs to incurring safety, if comfort is part of your magical need, include comfrey.

Prosperity: The vibration of comfort will bring security and ease to any financial situation. Comfrey has a dual magic of bringing luck in risky ventures where you are gambling with your success.

Protection: Comfrey's protection energy starts with relieving stress, creating comfort in your environment, and then ensuring safety. Use comfrey for protection and an easy journey in your travel spells.

Love: Spells to resolve trouble in any relationship need comfrey's energy of peace and ease.

Clearing: Comfrey's energy can transform and release old, pent-up emotions that may be causing discomfort and dis-ease.

Healing: The healing process is greatly benefited by comfrey's ability to calm down a troubled mind and spirit.

COPAL

Clearing, Healing

Copal resin opens your connection to the divine, your ancestry, and helpful spirits. It does this by purifying your energy, clearing it of what keeps you stuck in negative thought patterns. This is a potent resin, so a little goes a long way.

Prosperity: Copal's vibration brings the energizing positive energy that attracts abundance. When requested, this energy can be inspirational and open you to new opportunities. The grounding energies of copal can also be used to clear your blocks to the flow of abundance in your life.

Protection: Add copal to your protection spells to raise the vibration of your space, purifying it and bringing in balanced energy.

Love: When arguments and chaotic energy are harming your relationships, add copal to your spell to invite in warm, loving energy. This is also useful to clear away stagnant energy and bring back loving passion to a relationship.

Clearing: Copal's main purpose is to purify and lift the heavy negative energy that prevents your connection to the earth and the divine. Keep this resin or incense on hand to set up your space before any spell.

Healing: The ancient Aztecs called copal the blood of the tree and considered it a sacred healing compound. It is very grounding and elevating at the same time, bringing your energy into balance. Add copal to your healing spells to dissipate the energy that can contribute to anxiety and panic. The vibration of copal supports the strength of spirit needed to make positive change in your life.

CORIANDER

Prosperity, Love

Coriander helps you get comfortable in your own skin and brings the confidence needed to find your own divine voice.

Prosperity: Use coriander in prosperity spells where you need to ask for something—job interviews, sales calls, loans. It will lift fears around asking for what you want and inspire interest in the other party.

Protection: Coriander's protective vibration is perfect for the home, bringing peace and security.

Love: If you are casting a spell to heat up the lust in your life, add coriander. It works by helping all parties become comfortable and confident in enjoying each other in a mutually agreeable way. It is also an excellent ingredient for spells that ease conflict in the home.

Clearing: Coriander clears the fears around interaction with others, helping you find the confidence to use your voice in uncomfortable situations.

Healing: Using coriander in spells helps you get comfortable in your own skin and build confidence. This healing vibration opens you up to seeing your destiny and soul's purpose.

CUMIN

Prosperity

Cumin is the unsung ingredient in many savory recipes; something is just not right if it's missing. Magically, it has the same effect, bringing all ingredients together in harmony.

Prosperity: Cumin was at one time used as currency. Adding this prosperous energy to any spell brings wealth and hidden resources.

Protection: Use cumin if there are mischievous or harmful spirits around, as it will drive them out. Cumin also protects from loss and theft.

Love: Cumin has the reputation for promoting fidelity and lust in a relationship—is this the missing ingredient you need?

Clearing: Cumin is a good herb to clear out general negativity.

Healing: Cumin is purported to bring peace of mind, making it an easy addition to stress-busting spells.

CYPRESS

Protection, Clearing

Death, resurrection, and reincarnation are the core energies of cypress. Used to clear unending grief, cypress helps us through our personal transformations into a higher spiritual calling.

Prosperity: Use cypress when you are recovering from a devastating loss. It will lift your grief and ease your mind, helping you move forward to recovery.

Protection: Add cypress to your protection blend to prevent you from absorbing the grief and overwhelming emotions of others.

Love: Use cypress in spells to recover from a breakup or in cut and clear spells to help you move through the feelings of loss and prevent you from backtracking.

Clearing: Cypress's vibration simply moves overwhelming grief out of your body and aura, releasing it totally. This is also very useful in breaking a habit and letting go of past behaviors.

Healing: Cypress is uplifting, allow you to once again connect to your inner strength.

DAMIANA

Love

Known as *the* love and lust herb, damiana does not disappoint. Any aphrodisiac calls for this herb.

Prosperity: Damiana can be sparingly used for luck and swaying people to your side. (Be careful that they don't get a crush on you, though.)

Protection: A twist on the use of damiana is to protect you from being lonely.

Love: This is where damiana shines. Love, lust, a better sex life, drawing a lover closer, having good luck in love matters, increasing sexual prowess, and overall making your life a little steamier between the sheets and out of bed—damiana does it all.

Clearing: Damiana naturally clears fears around love and sexuality.

Healing: Interestingly, when asked and directed, damiana's energy can ease nervous tension and heightens psychic awareness.

DANDELION

Prosperity, Clearing

Harvest those dandelions before they are sprayed! This plant is very useful in psychic pursuits, among other things.

Prosperity: Add dandelion in your wish fulfillment spells. It is also very useful when you need to move through a creative block that is preventing your financial gain.

Protection: Grab your dried dandies and add them to a hex-breaking spell and protection blend. The lion part of the herb brings bravery and courage.

Love: Use dandelions to send psychic messages to loved ones and inspire a return connection.

Clearing: Dandelion's vibration clears the psychic centers as well as confusing thoughts.

Healing: Helpful spirits are drawn to the energy of the dandelion. They bring happiness, joy, and playful energy. Use dandelion to boost your creative process and bring in the sun energy to burn through blocks.

DATES AND FIGS

Prosperity, Love

Yes, these are two different plants, but they energetically hold a similar energy of bringing prosperity and fertility.

Prosperity: Prosperity, fertility, abundance, and joy are drawn by the vibration of dates and figs.

Protection: Both dates and figs in the home are protection against going hungry.

Love: Sacred to the gods of lust and play, dates and figs are the fruits of joy and remind us of the sweetness of life. Use these in love and lust charms to release any frigidness.

Clearing: The energy of these fruits pushes out fears around poverty and lack.

Healing: Use dates and figs in your spell to gift yourself with the stability you need to prosper and grow into your destiny.

DILL WEED

Prosperity, Protection

No, this is not an alternative to swearing at your brother. Dill weed is a must-have in your magical pantry for its vibration of protection, generosity, and good fortune.

Prosperity: Dill weed is very generous in its energy, and its good fortune grows in strength when shared. Add this to your success spells when you need strength of mind.

Protection: Dill weed is protective of infants and children. When used in protection spells,

it drives out evil, protects against the evil eye, and brings divine blessings.

Love: Use dill weed in your spell to create a bit of irresistible charm and lust.

Clearing: When you need to clear the confusion and make a differentiation between fantasy and reality, add dill weed to your spell.

Healing: The clarity, inner strength, and mental acuity brought with the vibration of dill weed make it a powerful addition to any healing spell.

DRAGON'S BLOOD

Prosperity, Protection, Healing

Dragon's blood, a resin from the fruit of the sangre de drago tree found in South America, Indonesia, and the Canary Islands, has a vibration of balance and harmony that heals and empowers.

Prosperity: Dragon's blood increases the power of any magical spell as it attunes your emotions and energy to your intention.

Protection: A ward against evil, dragon's blood can clear spiritual infestations.

Love: Use dragon's blood in reconciliation spells, drawing your lover back to fall in lust with you all over again.

Clearing: The scent of dragon's blood can calm a troubled mind and help you slip into a meditative state.

Healing: Dragon's blood is a vibration of balance and harmony. It connects you to the creative forces of the universe to heal and empower.

EUCALYPTUS

Protection, Clearing

Eucalyptus is one of my favorites for clearing the energy and hooks from others. It is an excellent ward against unwanted energy.

Prosperity: Use it to clear away any attacks on your abundance and success.

Protection: Eucalyptus is one of the first choices for protection. It works by powering up your will and resolve so you repel the harmful energy of others and any of your own inner sabotage.

Love: Add this in love spells to prevent unwanted influence.

Clearing: Eucalyptus is the herb and oil you want in every spell to spiritually cleanse you of others' energies and uncross yourself.

Healing: The healing powers of eucalyptus work to lift your spirit by cleaning you of the con-gestion of other people's energy. It helps lift oppressive stress and leaves a calm centered-ness in its wake.

EVERGREENS (FIR AND PINE)

Prosperity, Protection, Healing

The magic of an evergreen is at your fingertips whenever you need it. It is a promise that the wisdom of the ages is accessible to you.

Prosperity: The evergreen vibration is a money magnet and helps maintain your prosperity. It is known for its use in manifestation spells as it gives you permission for your wishes to manifest.

Protection: Use an evergreen in your protection spell to help build a fortress of strength and confidence.

Love: Evergreen in the home brings joy and peace to the house and promotes the longev-ity of a relationship.

Clearing: Fir, pine, and all evergreens help lift the spirit and clear it of the hooks, drains, and agendas that others may have imposed upon you.

Healing: Fir is known as a tree of life. Great wisdom and divinity are accessed through its energy. All evergreens are great for ancestral work.

FENNEL

Protection, Healing

Secrecy, perseverance, and strength of spirit are brought to you by the vibrations of fennel.

Prosperity: Add fennel to your spell to help you get through tough times by bringing in luck, grace, and balanced emotions.

Protection: Fennel's energy will face down any danger, legal matters, and negativity thrown at you. Use fennel to keep your secrets and privacy. It will also "out" those who are harm-ing others in secret.

Love: Fennel strengthens the heart and balances emotions. Use this when creating spells to strengthen your marriage or partnership.

Clearing: Fennel's vibration will clear out the hooks and drains of others.

Healing: When you are riding the roller coaster of drama, fennel will bring your spiritual energy back to balance and help you find your inner power.

FIVE FINGER GRASS (CINQUEFOIL)

Prosperity

If luck and favor will bring you success, five finger grass is your herb.

Prosperity: Five finger grass is your go-to for spells that involve anything that is gained by luck or favor. Overall, the vibration of five finger grass will help manifest your dreams.

Protection: Ward off evil, uncross, remove jinxes, and travel safely when you infuse five finger grass in your spell.

Love: To win the favor or attention of others with your spell, add in five finger grass.

Clearing: Include this grass in your cleansing baths and spells.

Healing: Use five finger grass to awaken feminine intuition.

FRANKINCENSE

Protection, Clearing, Healing

All major religions use frankincense resin to consecrate their sacred buildings and invite the divine into their congregation. They learned this from the ancient pagans who were already aware of frankincense's vibration and power.

Prosperity: Frankincense brings the luck and strength of spirit that promote a blessed and successful life.

Protection: Frankincense releases a powerful vibration that clears negativity in energy and spirit. Use it to purify and consecrate your sacred space.

Love: Frankincense's vibration works to clear you of obsessions around relationships that are not in your best interest. It will help cut the ties and unfulfilled hopes that bind you to the past.

Clearing: The vibration of frankincense clears fear, stress, depression, and tension, allowing you to raise your spiritual connection to the divine.

Healing: Frankincense invites in divine blessings that will lift depression and soothe the spirit.

GARLIC

Protection

More than a repellent of vampires and first dates, garlic is a very protective addition to your spell.

Prosperity: Use garlic to protect investments and financial risks. It will help you with confidence in situations where your risk is sound.

Protection: Use garlic in overall general protection. It clears negative influences and brings courage, especially in potentially catastrophic situations. It keeps out robbers and thieves.

Love: The vibration of garlic is helpful in keeping evil and envy away from new relationships. Ironically, it is reported to induce lust.

Clearing: Garlic clears negative energy and influence.

Healing: Garlic is well known for absorbing and guarding against diseases.

GERANIUM

Protection, Clearing
Geranium's protective energy is specific for the home and marriage.

Prosperity: Not known for its general qualities of prosperity, geranium could be used to protect family property and wealth.

Protection: Use all types of geranium for general protection, specifically when someone is emotionally exhausted from continual abuse.

Love: Geranium is sacred to Hymenaios, the god of marriage. Use it to bless and ensure a strong and loving marriage. A vow said under the blessing of geranium will not be broken.

Clearing: Red geraniums are known for their cleansing and healing energy.

Healing: If emotional exhaustion and depression after trauma are affecting your energy, geranium is your magical go-to.

GINGER

Prosperity, Protection, Love, Healing
This powerful root is a must for your magical cupboard. It is very easy to get fresh and will power up any spell you are casting, while creating protection while you are doing it.

Prosperity: The vibrations of ginger attract money and triple the power of any money magic spell. The heat and speed of ginger's energy bring luck with it.

Protection: Ginger has big, fiery protection energy, burning away any negative intent sent your way. It is great for protection against bad dreams and evil spirits.

Love: Ginger heats up a love spell, increasing sexual desire and potency. You can also direct ginger to open up the Akashic records to call your destined healthy love match in this lifetime.

Clearing: Ginger, when combined with healing herbs, can be used to energetically draw out sickness. In its protective energy, it will clear out any negativity that is affecting you.

Healing: Ginger is well known for its own healing qualities as well its reputation to increase the magical potency of anything it is combined with. It also powers up intuition, courage, and strength of character.

HONEYSUCKLE

Prosperity, Love
Honeysuckle's energy is filled with hope, fulfill-ment, resolve, and psychic clarity.

Prosperity: Honeysuckle's energy is a natural draw to prosperity. It invites the sweetness of life to take root in *your* life. It will bring clarity to your situation so you can see a way forward and find some relief. Honeysuckle also helps to strengthen the resolve needed to fulfill your goals, increases your psychic awareness and spiritual insight, and brings clarity and understanding to any clairvoyant images you receive.

Protection: Not a specifically protective flower, honeysuckle will, however, strengthen your resolve for fulfilling your goals.

Love: Honeysuckle gives you insight into the connection you have with others and helps you see what your future together will hold. Use honeysuckle in your love spells to invite sweetness into your relationship.

Clearing: Use honeysuckle in any manifesting spell to clear confusion and bring clarity.

Healing: Honeysuckle is a manifestation flower. Its vibration strengthens your resolve, boosts psychic awareness, and provides clarity to the information you receive.

HYSSOP

Clearing
Hyssop is a favorite of witches to protect and clear before doing any magic.

Prosperity: Hyssop's protective vibration will clear jealousy and sabotage from your mate-rial success.

Protection: The main purpose of hyssop is protection, specifically for your home. Use it to keep negative intentions, thieves, and saboteurs away.

Love: Use hyssop in spells where you are creat-ing a state of peace and security for all who reside there.

Clearing: Hyssop oil is perfect for spells that purify, drive away evil, and lift one to a higher spiritual purpose. Use with rue to create a preritual anointing oil and to cleanse magical tools.

Healing: Healers wear this to protect them in the healing process to avoid attachments from their clients.

IRISH MOSS (SEA MOSS)

Prosperity
I am very excited to introduce you to the energy of Irish moss. This sea moss brings in a tide of prosperity.

Prosperity: Irish moss's energy increases luck and a steady flow of money. It brings steady *paying* customers.

Protection: Irish moss is protective of your financial situation and in travel, especially for business.

Love: Not a love herb per se, Irish moss can be used in relationship or community spells to ease any financial stress that is causing discord.

Clearing: Irish moss is a red alga from the Atlantic, and its energy can help you move with the energy around you, removing any resistance and rigidity that may be draining you.

Healing: Magically Irish moss can be used to keep you flexible in attitude to be able to see the opportunities in front of you.

JASMINE

Love, Healing

Jasmine is a gift from the goddess; it is said that she smiled upon all of life and turned that smile into jasmine.

Prosperity: Jasmine's energy is a dream come true. Specify your intent and desired outcome, and she will make it happen.

Protection: Jasmine promotes a sense of well-being, and from this state of balance you can find confidence and a sense of self that become protective.

Love: Jasmine is a must for your love spells: she warms your heart and attracts all levels of nurturing love, whether physical, emotional, or spiritual. No matter your sexual identity, jasmine attracts females and induces sexual desire.

Clearing: Jasmine's vibration of love and fulfillment naturally lifts spirits and clears the emotional states that keep you depressed and anxiety-ridden.

Healing: Jasmine's vibration brings a level of peace to the spirit where your walls, blockages, and self-sabotage start to fall away. This space is quickly filtered so only positive energy remains.

JUNIPER

Protection, Healing

Juniper has some unique magical vibrations of protection from external and internal negativity. It strengthens your resolve and personal will.

Prosperity: Use juniper in your money spell when you are reaching for a goal as it brings the strength and discipline to follow through.

Protection: Juniper's energy is protective of the home to guard against attacks, theft, and sickness. It also protects you from curses, hexes, and your own self-sabotage. It's particular protective vibration comes from an increase in your psychic powers to be able to see and break the negativity in your life.

Love: Juniper is said to increase love's potency.

Clearing: The clearing powers of juniper work hand in hand with its protective powers to remove hexes and curses and clear away self-sabotage.

Healing: Juniper, surprisingly, is a self-care herb as it strengthens your dedication to taking care of yourself. This resolve is restorative to body, mind, and spirit.

LAVENDER

Love
Lavender's vibration brings unconditional love and instills a desire to return the love with compassion and respect.

Prosperity: Use lavender in prosperity spells that need extra confidence and peace with the outcome.

Protection: Lavender's love vibration protects against envy, cruelty, abuse, infidelity, and sorrow.

Love: Lavender is the protector of love and belongs in every love spell you wish to put it in. It invites warm feelings of compassion, kindness, nurturing, and the inner confidence of self-love. These feelings are a natural magnet when you are attracting a love interest or deepening love.

Clearing: Lavender's love vibrations will induce restful, healing sleep and calm a storm of emotions. It also helps cleanse the spirit of the evil eye.

Healing: Lavender's vibration makes all sorrow depart so that joys can be fully present and empower healing.

LEMON BALM

Prosperity, Clearing
Lemon balm is the bad luck buster.

Prosperity: Lemon balm is great for prosperity spells as it clears away bad luck, allowing good luck a place to take root. Even if that bad luck comes from your own nervousness and anxiety, lemon balm will override it all to let your intention manifest.

Protection: Clears the unfavorable condition that is troubling you and keeps it from breaking your confidence in the protection magic you have cast.

Love: Lemon balm attracts love by adding the energy to be more attractive and desirable.

Clearing: Lemon balm is the bad luck buster, clearing crossed energy away from you. It will also clear the nervousness, anxiety, and clouded mind that create crossed conditions.

Healing: Lemon balm's vibration breaks bad conditions in any form and promotes good health in mind, emotion, and body. It brings confidence in your contribution to the world.

LEMONGRASS

Prosperity, Clearing
Lemongrass's vibration is transformative, turning negative energy into positive. It brings out the truth of a situation and helps you see through lies.

Prosperity: Lemongrass's energy opens the road to new prospects and adds a boost of energy to any of your magical intentions. It is a bad luck buster and will change your luck to good.

Protection: Lemongrass will protect your energy when you are vulnerable or stressed. It does this by transforming negative energy into positive and compelling the truth of a situation.

Love: Lemongrass does us the favor of clearing away the expectations and lies we tell ourselves so that we can see the true potential in a relationship. It can clear away the fantasy or idea we create around the relationship we really want. It also increases lust.

Clearing: Lemongrass's transformative vibration clears away bad luck, evil intent, and the lies that you have been told.

Healing: Lemongrass is essential to the preparation of any magical journey. It will protect your energy while your psychic centers are opened and your awareness increased.

MARJORAM

Love

Marjoram vibrates the peace of a loving marriage or partnership.

Prosperity: If you have a partnership that affects your prosperity, marjoram strengthens that commitment and helps ease fears around it.

Protection: Marjoram has a natural vibration that is protective of the household.

Love: Marjoram is the herb of love and marriage. It vibrates peace and comfort, helping the love within a marriage to deepen on every level.

Clearing: Marjoram's peaceful, loving vibration is helpful in times of sorrow and grief, reconnecting you to the cycle of life to let go of the sorrow.

Healing: Marjoram's vibration helps heal rifts in relationships and teaches you how to embrace your own worthiness of love.

MINTS (PEPPERMINT, SPEARMINT, WINTERGREEN, AND COMMON MINT)

Love

All mint variations have the magic to clear out the negative and obsessive energy that can reside in the mind and in your environment.

Prosperity: Mint's energy attracts and protects money. Is it known to grant good fortune.

Protection: The mind and spirit are protected by mint energy. It clears and protects the mind of obsessive thoughts and will safeguard you while sleeping.

Love: The mint family will help clear obsessions in love matters so you can find true and real love. It will, when directed, induce lust.

Clearing: Mint's vibration pulls out negative energy from surfaces as well as the environment. Used in clearing spells, it removes hexes and curses and removes the energetic hooks left by controlling people.

Healing: Mint's visionary properties bring out what was hidden to the conscious mind, removing what may have been blocking your visualizations and connection with the divine.

Used in self-purification rituals, mint will clear your mind, calm your nerves, and lift your spirit. Even a cup of peppermint tea can lift your spirits, clear your mind, and awaken psychic visions.

MUGWORT

Healing

Mugwort is a visionary herb. Its energy powers up your psychic abilities and protects them from negative energy as they grow.

Prosperity: Although it is not a prosperity herb, you can use mugwort in spells where you are creating a vision for your future.

Protection: Mugwort's visionary energy has the additional benefit of being protective against negative spirits and darker forces while allying you with benevolent spirits. Use in spells that protect children, as they are naturally open conduits of psychic energy.

Love: Mugwort's vibration helps you to see through gaslighting and maintain your boundaries.

Clearing: Mugwort is a natural cleanser of psychic residue and any wayward spirits that are trying to attach to you.

Healing: Mugwort's energy is effective in seeking dream visions and prophetic visions and increasing psychic awareness.

MUSTARD SEEDS

Protection, Prosperity, Healing

"If you have faith as small as a mustard seed . . . ," the Bible tells us you will be able to move mountains. The magic of mustard seed is to build confidence and connection to the divine.

Prosperity: Mustard seeds vibrate big energy around confidence and strength of character. When that is present in your prosperity spells, you will be successful and lucky.

Protection: This vibration automatically wards off evil and keeps the supernatural from entering your home. Mustard seed energy protects your voice, especially when performing or speaking about difficult subjects.

Love: Mustard seed is rumored to enhance the male sexual nature . . . Another offshoot of the confidence mustard seeds bring?

Clearing: Mustard seeds are more of a drawing vibration than a clearing one. However, if needed, use them to bring confidence, strength, and faith when doing spiritual cleansing work.

Healing: Mustard seeds have an energy that aligns with good health. It is an herb that was sacred to surgeons and helps bring a mastery to healing and faith in outcomes.

MYRRH

Prosperity, Protection, Healing

The vibration of myrrh awakens and expands your awareness of the spiritual connection to all of life.

Prosperity: Myrrh calms fears and instills confidence in your future. This is very helpful in prosperity spells that are uncertain and need you to brave a new path. Myrrh is the earth of the "heaven and earth" manifestation pair of frankincense and myrrh. It creates a prosperous and stable foundation for your dreams to manifest upon.

Protection: Myrrh's vibration is cleansing and protective. It raises the vibration to invite in divine blessings, thus consecrating the space and tools you are working with and protecting them from outside influence.

Love: Used in a reconciliation spell, myrrh's energy will bring warmth, peace, and sensuality.

Clearing: When you use myrrh to bring peace and confidence, its vibration will naturally clear the fears generated from sorrow, abuse, and tragedy. Myrrh helps people to understand and work through transition, death, and grieving. Use the incense smoke to consecrate your magical objects, talismans, and tools, for myrrh increases the power of any other essence with which you work and purifies the area you are working in to raise the vibration.

Healing: Myrrh is the essence the phoenix is born from, so use this energy when you are needing to start over and find a new path. Myrrh's vibration brings an understanding of your destiny and how you fit into the great workings of the universe. It does this by gently growing your spiritual wisdom to help you understand how to apply this knowledge in everyday life.

NETTLES

Protection, Clearing

The vibration of nettles will dispel psychic attacks, curses, and negative spirits and return them to sender. It will clear hexes, jinxes, curses, and crossed conditions.

Prosperity: Nettles won't draw prosperity, but will clear hexes, curses, and crossed conditions around your prosperity, in turn strengthening your magic.

Protection: Nettles' protective vibration helps to keep ghosts away and strengthen your protective barriers when hexes and negative intents are thrown your way.

Love: Nettles are not a love-drawing herb, but they can be used in spells to help you overcome deep-seated fears around relationships.

Clearing: Nettles' vibration, when directed, is powerful return-to-sender magic. Be careful in case you are the cause of your own negativity. Nettles are best used to clear curses and hexes and the fears they triggered.

Healing: Nettles' vibration can help uncover and clear deep-seated family curses or legacies. They are also useful in spells to clear entities that are hooked into your energy.

NIGHTSHADE (BELLADONNA)

Protection, Clearing

First things first: nightshade/belladonna is *poisonous*! Nightshade has the reputation as a cursing herb, but its strong protective quality proves the adage of "what can curse can heal, and what can heal can curse." Potatoes, tomatoes, sweet and hot peppers, eggplants, tomatillos, pepinos, pimentos, paprika, and cayenne are all in the nightshade family; if you can't find a bit of nightshade for your spell, pinch some green off of one of these.

Prosperity: Nightshade's energy is ripe with the magic needed to manifest of your intent. Use it in spells where you need to start over and clear the grief and fears of your past experience.

Protection: Nightshade is very protective of homes. Its presence will catch negative energies thrown at you and reverse them. It is also effective in spells to protect your reputation and how other people see you.

Love: *Belladonna* means "beautiful lady," making it useful in spells to build your self-image and confidence. Inversely, its vibration will ease the grief and ugliness of betrayal.

Clearing: A main ingredient in a reverse the curse spell, nightshade's big vibration breaks hexes—and can hex as well—and clears the fallout from them.

Healing: In rituals for the dead to help a loved one move on to the next realm, nightshade's energy is a beautiful addition. You can also use her vibrations in spells to cut away the old and begin a new life.

NUTMEG

Prosperity, Healing

Nutmeg is a versatile spice that has a mutable vibration that can be aligned with what you intend to manifest. A little goes a long way with nutmeg. A small amount is balancing, and too much can take you into the fantasy of an ideal that is not possible.

The energy of nutmeg keeps things moving and brings you into balance with what you wish to have happen; in other words, it helps your vibration match what it is you want to manifest. Traditionally, nutmeg's charms were worn for luck and to ward off sickness. If you want love, bake nutmeg into a sweet and feed it to the one you are interested in. No matter what your spell or magic, nutmeg increases your psychic awareness.

In aromatherapy, a little nutmeg goes a long way as a remedy for many mental ailments such as anxiety, depression, nervousness, and neurotic symptoms.

Prosperity: The energy of nutmeg keeps things moving toward your goal. Its vibration helps you shift your vibration to match what you are manifesting.

Protection: Use it in protection spells to ward off sickness and disillusionment.

Love: Apply nutmeg in your love spell to have your interest returned to you.

Clearing: Nutmeg's powers of manifestation naturally relieve you of anxiety, depression, and nervousness, replacing them with confidence. Too much nutmeg in your spell will increase your anxiety-ridden feelings.

Healing: No matter what your spell or magic, nutmeg increases your psychic awareness and helps you see what is next in your spiritual evolution.

OAKMOSS

Prosperity

Oakmoss's vibration is expansive, helping any magic you're attempting to grow bigger and move faster. Its need for symbiosis in nature brings the energy of cooperation and the understanding of how the smallest change can have a big impact on your environment.

Prosperity: Oakmoss has big luck and money energy. Prosperity spells where you need all factors to fall in line in your favor will benefit from oakmoss as will spells where you need to grow bigger and make a big financial score.

Protection: Oakmoss is very grounding. This vibration, combined with the vibration to sense subtle changes in your environment, makes oakmoss a good addition to a magical early warning system for your protection.

Love: Oakmoss, first and foremost, will help build your relationship with nature. Its vibration will tune in to the messages from nature spirits and the goddesses of earth. Oakmoss in love spells will help you find an understanding of how the actions of one affect both. Its scent heightens erotic feelings and can pull in the wild, unpredictable energy of Pan.

Clearing: The grounding vibration of oakmoss brings a calm balance that puts you in an emotional place where you can let go of the past.

Healing: Oakmoss can be added to healing spells to calm fears and speed the healing process.

ORANGE BLOSSOM (NEROLI)

Prosperity, Love, Clearing

Neroli's magic lies in its ability to banish negative thoughts; it is almost miraculous in its vibration. This vibration is helpful in all branches of the Magic 5.

Prosperity: Orange blossom's vibration of positive energy is a natural money draw. When you clear negative thoughts, your spirit is lifted, and your belief in your magic is unstoppable.

Protection: Orange blossom's ability to calm the mind and clear it of negative influence is the precursor to powerful protection spells.

Love: The warm energy of orange blossom helps clear and heal fears around sexuality. When used in a love spell, it will warm all parties to the idea of connecting.

Clearing: Orange blossom helps to banish negative thoughts, clearing overwhelming emotional upsets, shock, anxiety, and depression.

Healing: Orange blossom's spirit-lifting vibration is naturally healing. It will bring thoughts and emotions back into balance and clear the spiritual patterns that are draining your vital energy.

ORRIS ROOT (IRIS)

Love, Healing
Orris root (iris) is the vibration of the divine feminine. All issues dealing with women and feminine energy are benefited by orris root.

Prosperity: The vibration of orris root brings faith in yourself and the wisdom of the divine. Use in prosperity spells that need faith and courage for what you are about to embark upon.

Protection: Use orris root in protection spells to keep the negative or evil intent of others away from you. Orris root brings courage and valor to your energy, giving an additional boost to your magic.

Love: Orris root is sacred to the goddess in all her forms, including love. Add orris root to your love-drawing spells, especially when you are attracting a man. This root also energizes the qualities of a long-lasting loving relationship and all general love qualities like passion, romance, and marriage.

Clearing: The iris is a funeral flower whose vibration helps souls pass to the next realm. Use orris root in spells to clear spirits and haunts.

Healing: Orris root is sacred to the goddess in all her forms. Use this herb when seeking a deeper connection to the divine, asking for her guidance and divine blessings.

PARSLEY

Prosperity, Protection
Parsley's magical energy is not limited to the garnish on your plate. This is an herb that gives you a boost in attaining your goal and transcending death of any kind—death of spirit, ideas, relationships, future goals, and so on.

Prosperity: Use the speedy vibration of success and victory that parsley brings in your prosperity spells. Parsley is also known to be highly effective in landlord and real estate transactions.

Protection: Parsley in your protection spell will prevent mental manipulation and guard against misfortune. It was originally placed on plates of food to protect against contamination.

Love: As a love herb, parsley attracts a romantic partner.

Clearing: Use the vibration of parsley to clear your mind of manipulation and gaslighting. This will bring confidence in your own decisions.

Healing: As an herb used to transcend death, parsley helps you overcome the loss and grief of unwanted endings. The energy of parsley also creates a clear channel when communicating with the divine.

PATCHOULI

Prosperity, Love, Healing

Patchouli has a very earthy vibration that connects the body with the force of creation. Its energy shows you how to cocreate with all of life.

Prosperity: Patchouli's vibration connects your body to creative forces including fertility that help you manifest money and other resources.

Protection: The grounding and calming energy of patchouli helps you get back into the body in times of stress and focus your energy on a protective goal.

Love: Patchouli's grounded energy helps you be yourself and in alignment with your higher calling; this attracts partners that align with you. Sexual desire can be aroused when patchouli's essence is around as it releases anxiety around sex, promotes lust, and stimulates passion between two people.

Clearing: Patchouli's energy releases anxiety around expressing your passion.

Healing: Patchouli's vibration helps you step into your true, higher self. This awareness assists you in seeing who brings cooperation and partnership to your life. It also connects you with the cocreative powers of life and charges up divine inspiration.

PENNYROYAL

Prosperity, Protection, Clearing

Pennyroyal's quiet, calm vibration opens your senses to the cycles with any situation. This helps with prosperity, protection, and relationship challenges.

Prosperity: Pennyroyal's vibration is a calm strength that allows you to see the cycles of life, making this an excellent choice in spells for successful business deals.

Protection: Pennyroyal's energy is very protective; it wards off the evil eye, breaks jinxes, and is particularly attuned to the family and marriage.

Love: For spells to quiet marital arguments, use pennyroyal. It instills overall tranquility in the home and draws good luck for the family.

Clearing: Pennyroyal's vibration clears the evil and breaks jinxes, especially for family and love matters.

Healing: Sacred to Demeter, pennyroyal imparts the wisdom and power of life and rebirth. It also strengthens the body when you have emotional weariness.

PEONY

Love, Clearing

Peony is passion, protection, and clarity. It is used in love spells, to call guardian protectors, and to make hard decisions.

Prosperity: When you have difficult choices involving prosperity, peony seeds help bring the clarity needed to decide.

Protection: Peony's love vibration makes it impossible for evil or negativity to enter. It calls to your guardian protectors for spirit, body, and soul.

Love: Peony's vibration is passionate, filling the spirit with love, releasing fears, and inspiring lust and sensuality.

Clearing: Peony's vibration helps clear the mind when you are faced with difficult decisions.

Healing: The guardian-calling energy of peony can be directed to call spirits that heal through love.

PEPPERCORN

Protection, Clearing

Peppercorn's energy increases the effect of anything it is combined with. It is also commonly used in protection spells and to break and clear hexes. (It can be used to hex as well.)

Prosperity: Peppercorn has a grounding and stabilizing vibration that will heighten your awareness of the circumstances around you. When you see what is going on, you can make better decisions around your financial needs.

Protection: Peppercorn's badass vibrations protect you from energies thrown at you

to create sabotage and chaos—the evil eye, curses, hexes, bad-mouthing. It will prevent unwanted people from visiting physically, spiritually, or virtually.

Love: Peppercorn oil is an interesting addition to heat up lust spells and bring confidence in matters of love.

Clearing: Peppercorn's energy frees the mind of envious thoughts—from you or directed at you. Use peppercorn in spells to break hexes.

Healing: Not a specifically healing herb, a small amount of peppercorn can ground and stabilize you as well as speed up the healing process. Larger amounts can become irritating.

POPPY

Prosperity, Love, Healing

Poppy flowers vibrate good luck in love, money, and health matters. Poppy seeds can sow confusion.

Prosperity: Poppy flowers vibrate good luck. Use them in financial and property spells to be in the right place at the right time. Poppy also brings the energy of fertility into your projects and goals.

Protection: Use poppy seeds in spells where you need to confuse who is attacking you and cloud their ability to even think about you.

Love: Poppy flowers bring good luck energy for love spells. It can help you dream or vision a new love.

Clearing: When directed, poppy can bring clarity to a situation or create confusion.

Healing: Poppy's vibration affects the mind and the way we process emotions. Use the energy of the flowers and seeds together to bring a mental and emotional balance.

ROSE

Love, Protection, Healing
Rose is the vibration of peace and tranquility, turning thoughts to love and calming conflict.

Prosperity: Rose's energy of confidence and its attractiveness to fairies and good spirits make it an excellent addition in fast luck spells.

Protection: The peace and calm that rose brings banish doubt, raise confidence, and create a powerful protective energy. Rose has been used traditionally as incense or as a dried flower to keep secret all that was said in the room.

Love: Rose's vibration is a powerful aphrodisiac. Rose brings love and romance and draws love of all kinds to a spell. Rose's energy inspires passion and, when directed, will bring back a lost love.

Clearing: The peace and calm that rose vibrates can banish depression and heal heartbreak.

Healing: Rose has a lovely overall healing vibration.

ROSEMARY

Clearing, Protection
Rosemary is in the top five of my favorite magical herbs. It is cleansing, protective, and mind-expanding.

Prosperity: Rosemary's energy can make you memorable—put it in a new job spell and all other candidates will pale in comparison to the impression you make. As a feminine herb, rosemary's vibration helps women find and embrace their personal power and bring it into balance for leadership and responsibility.

Protection: The protective energy of rosemary will safeguard you from thieves, rid the place of negativity, and shelter everyone within against dis-ease.

Love: The vibration of rosemary is useful in love and marriage spells. It will power up your magic, clear negative memories, and bring longevity to the relationship.

Clearing: Rosemary's magic is around remembrance through keeping the mind clear. Its cleansing and purification vibrations are perfect when you are on spiritual overload.

Healing: Rosemary's vibration keeps you clear and balanced when you are pursuing spiritual growth. Use for inspiration spells to apply what you know to a new idea. Add it to your ancestor offerings and in dream magic to remember them. Rosemary's energy is excellent in spells to clear grief, allowing one to fondly remember loved ones who have died while releasing the overwhelming and irrational emotions.

ROWAN

Protection
The deva of rowan is very protective, wise, and sacred to the goddess.

Prosperity: Use rowan in spells to protect you from experiences of loss and stress.

Protection: Rowan's vibration is very protective, especially in the home. Use it in spells to protect from evil and negative energies, as a countermeasure for any magical attack, and to add the blessings of the goddess to your protection magic.

Love: Use rowan in spells where you are protecting and strengthening the family unit.

Clearing: Rowan's blessed and protective energy can help clear dis-ease.

Healing: Rowan is considered a sacred tree of life that we gain wisdom from. Its vibration increases psychic powers and works to heal a wounded spirit.

RUE

Protection
A favorite of the witches, rue's vibration is spiritually protective.

Prosperity: Use rue in spells where you are protecting your prosperity.

Protection: Add the vibration of rue to all of your protection spells, especially when you are performing magic or rituals. Rue will block any negative energy sent your way.

Love: Rue's energy in love spells will clear the mind of manipulation. It clears the mind in love issues, and it clears manipulative spells concerning love and relationships.

Clearing: Add rue to your house-clearing spells to get free of negativity. Rue is a powerful addition to hex- and curse-breaking spells to clear the spiritual hook of entities that accompanied them.

Healing: Rue's protective vibration can ward off illness and speed recovery.

SAFFRON/SAFFLOWER

Protection, Healing
Saffron's power as a magical herb has been known since antiquity. A little goes a long way to clear depressive energy and bring in the power of love.

Prosperity: Saffron's vibration is divine and brings blessings of magical power and fertility. Use it in prosperity spells where you are creating something new.

Protection: Saffron's energy increases the power of any spell. In your protection spells it will amp up your work.

Love: Saffron is a powerful love herb. Employ it in your love-drawing spells, especially when attracting a male lover.

Clearing: Saffron's golden-yellow vibration breaks up and clears depressive and oppressive energy.

Healing: Saffron's bright golden-yellow color connects you to the sacredness of all life.

Use this in spells that call to your divine to bring insight and awaken your innate magical powers.

SAGE

Prosperity, Clearing
A must-have for every magical cupboard, this cleansing, protective, abundant, loving, and healing herb hits all of the Magic 5.

Prosperity: We forget that sage has a very powerful prosperity vibration. Use this in spells to ensure secure finances, get a good job, or fulfill any deep wish that you have. Women in business are empowered by the vibrations of sage; it helps them hold their own in a world of men and embrace success. Single mothers benefit from using sage in spells that meet all the household financial and emotional needs.

Protection: Sage sets a barrier of protection around the user, keeping evil and negativity at bay.

Love: The wish-granting vibration of sage makes it an effective addition to love-drawing spells. Sage also gives strength to women, helping them see their worth, and healing issues around self-image and being attractive to others.

Clearing: Sage is the ultimate spiritual cleansing herb and must be used in every spell with this intent. It purifies your spiritual space as it cleanses your spirit of negativity and clears any evil or negative energy that is present.

Healing: The vibration of sage is the reason why the term was coined to mean wise advice. This energy brings wisdom and sagacity into a meeting of minds. Sage relieves mental and emotional stress and enhances wisdom so you can see your problems clearly.

SAINT-JOHN'S-WORT

Healing, Clearing
Tied to the energies of midsummer and the summer solstice, Saint-John's-wort brings happiness and connection to your own worth and power.

Prosperity: This herb brings an understanding of your true (usually underrated) value.

Protection: Use Saint-John's-wort in spells to drive away evil spirits and protect you from demons. Its vibration helps you conquer your

own inner demons by connecting you with your true purpose.

Love: The energy of Saint-John's-wort brings a cheer and happiness that naturally attract love and companionship.

Clearing: Use Saint-John's-wort to cleanse your home of negative energies and spirits.

Healing: The vibration of Saint-John's-wort helps one see their true value and inner strength. Use it in spells to bring the joy and happiness that will lift your spirit.

SANDALWOOD

Protection, Healing

As a sacred wood to many deities, it is near impossible for negativity to exist when sandalwood is present.

Prosperity: Sandalwood sends your wishes and prayers to the divine. It vibrates with the energy of cocreation and is perfect in spells where you are manifesting success.

Protection: When sandalwood is present, negativity is blocked, making this an excellent wood to add to protection and exorcism spells.

Love: Sandalwood brings confidence in all love and relationship matters. This is also an excellent addition to spells to smooth out and clear family arguments.

Clearing: Sandalwood's vibration deepens meditation by creating a solid connection with your higher power and pushing away limiting, negative, and oppressive energies.

Healing: Sandalwood raises energetic vibrations to a higher and more intense level of spirituality. It can help spirits cross the veil.

SASSAFRAS

Prosperity

Money, abundance, successful business, protecting investments—this is the businessperson's bark.

Prosperity: Sassafras's magic is almost solely dedicated to money—attracting it, healing emotional wounds around it, bringing clarity to business decisions, and steadily increasing business.

Protection: Use in spells that protect your investments.

Love: Sassafras attracts repeat customers and helps you build loyal relationships with them.

Clearing: Clears out stress around financial matters and brings a calm wisdom to your decisions.

Healing: The energy of sassafras is excellent in spells where your emotional wounds around money need to be addressed and healed.

SAVORY

Love, Healing

Savory is sacred to the god Pan and brings in the playful side of his energy.

Prosperity: Include savory in spells where you are needing energy and motivation.

Protection: Savory strengthens the mind through bringing joy and overall happiness.

Love: Savory's core energy is one of lust and play. Sacred to Pan and named after satyrs, this herb has warming energy that promotes laughter and joy. Savory can bring sexual drive into balance and help align the sexual needs of partners.

Clearing: The warm and playful energy of savory can clear out inhibitions to joy.

Healing: Overall joy is the outcome of savory—as well as abandon, laughter, and high energy.

TARRAGON

Protection

Tarragon's name means "little dragon." It is a very protective herb that is sacred to Lilith. It helps protect and heal in situations that are abusive.

Prosperity: Tarragon is wonderful for women in business as it brings confidence and protection from abusive situations.

Protection: Sacred to Lilith, tarragon protects women and children in abusive situations and helps them reclaim their strength and independence. Placed in a talisman, it also protects from future abuse.

Love: Use this herb in spells that empower women and bring self-assurance. Tarragon promotes compassion, love, and nurturing to and from your family while also helping you set boundaries.

Clearing: Include tarragon in spells to clear soul parts that were left behind by abusers. This is also a useful energy to have present when you are clearing trauma that can destroy your confidence.

Healing: Tarragon brings compassion for others and helps keep boundaries. For women who are caretakers it ensures they are also taking care of themselves.

THYME

Love, Healing

Thyme is an herb that thins the veil to other realms and dimensions. It brings a lighthearted approach to life.

Prosperity: Thyme lifts the drudgery of hard work and brings joy and luck to all you do. This energy creates a natural protection around your prosperity and finances.

Protection: A naturally protective herb as it is part of the mint and evergreen family. Thyme as a plant quickly spreads, creating a barrier to negative energy. This herb will also increase your courage and bravery in difficult situations.

Love: Use thyme to communicate or broadcast your romantic intentions. The energy of joy that thyme brings reminds you that first and foremost relationships are supposed to be enjoyable.

Clearing: Thyme relieves the unending seriousness of life and replaces it with joy, courage, and bravery.

Healing: Thyme connects you to other dimensions and realms, helping you communicate with the beings that reside there. Fairy folk, ancestors, and spirit guides are more accessible when thyme is present.

TURMERIC

Prosperity, Protection, Healing

Turmeric is my very good friend when it comes to managing the inflammation of my joints. It is a highly esteemed addition to many natural remedies, and this tells the tale of its magical energy.

Prosperity: Called the golden spice, turmeric goes into your prosperity spells to bring blessings, protection, and success. It helps you release the tension and stress that prevent you from seeing opportunity.

Protection: Use turmeric when creating a spell that protects your magical space. It is also very effective to protect you when you are traveling for business or work.

Love: Use the stress-relieving vibration of turmeric in love spells to open your eyes to the love that surrounds you.

Clearing: Turmeric is a beautiful addition to your purification spells. It clears out what was stuck and causes you pain. Is also helpful in keeping your memory clear.

Healing: This spice is used in many physical healing applications, making it a wonderful addition to healing spells. It will warm up your spirit and refill its energy as you cleanse.

UVA-URSI

Prosperity, Clearing, Healing

Uva-ursi's berries are the favorite of bears, giving it the alternate name of bearberry and the magic to increase the potency of any spell.

Prosperity: Straight up, uva-ursi will increase the power of any spell and is very rejuvenating.

Protection: Use it to bring protection in your psychic work.

Love: It clears the influence of others and your own obsessive thoughts, helping you see the truth of a relationship instead of what you want to be true.

Clearing: Uva-ursi clears your psychic energies.

Healing: Uva-ursi is a good choice to increase the potency of healing and visionary spells. It will bring protection to your psychic development as well as increase your ability.

VALERIAN

Clearing, Healing

Valium comes from valerian and its mellow calming energy. This is a distinctly stinky herb. A little goes a long way.

Prosperity: When you move into calm, mellow energy, the fears that would block your prosperity can't flourish. Put valerian in prosperity spells that need to overcome jealousy and personal fears.

Protection: Valerian loves to counter the evil eye and protect you from being crossed or hexed. It does this by keeping your energy calm and smooth so any negativity can't stick to you and maybe will be returned to sender.

Love: Valerian brings calm to troubled relationships, be they with a spouse, neighbor, business, family, or friends. Love spells that attract men can benefit from valerian, but be careful because this herb stinks.

Clearing: When the negativity of others becomes overwhelming, valerian can help clear out any jinx, hex, or evil eye. Its calming energy helps you let go of the anger that can keep this energy stuck on you.

Healing: The calming influence of valerian is a benefit to healing spells as it allows your energy to settle while you work on balancing it. It brings serenity and focus as you are preparing for a ritual.

VANILLA

Love

The vanilla bean, with its deep sweet essence, is the most popular scent and flavor in the world. Tap into its magical properties every day as you find its presence in your food and fragrances.

Prosperity: Vanilla helps you move from the vibration of lack to a vibration of abundance. It will lift your spirits and clear the mind when financial woes become depressing and overwhelming. Use it in confidence spells.

Protection: Use vanilla in protection spells to bring confidence and restore the energy that is being drained through the stress of safety issues. It also helps you transform through the experience and find the sweetness that life can bring.

Love: Vanilla's core magic is love, warming your emotions to feel the love around you and know you are deserving of it. Vanilla will hold this loving energy as you get used to feeling it. Vanilla is also a powerful ingredient in lust spells and particularly attractive to men. It inspires a loving, healthy relationship.

Clearing: Vanilla helps to clear depressed and despondent feelings by bringing in loving thoughts toward yourself and others.

Healing: Use vanilla in healing spells where you need to hold the vibration of loving thoughts when it feels impossible to connect to them. This is a powerful ingredient in spells that strengthen the mind and bring confidence.

VERVAIN

Clearing

Vervain is an herb that increases the magical properties of anything combined with it. It has a strengthening and expansive energy.

Prosperity: Vervain clears aways blocks to prosperity and powers up any spell.

Protection: Negative energies and entities that would attach to a practitioner as they work with spirits are cleared out by vervain. It will strengthen any protection spells and create a barrier against those who are envious and wish you harm, including any self-destructive behaviors.

Love: It increases the passion between two people and is used to draw love to you. It can be used to increase happiness in a marriage.

Clearing: Vervain clears negative entities and breaks any baneful spells or hexes that have been sent to you.

Healing: Vervain strengthens the mind and spirit while retaining all knowledge gained. Vervain calms the mind and expands dreaming and visualization skills.

WORMWOOD

Healing
A well-known visionary herb, wormwood brings calm and peace while dispelling great anger.

Prosperity: Wormwood helps you move past disappointments and into creative solutions.

Protection: It protects against bewitchment and unhealthy influence from another. It secures vehicles from accidents and keeps your travel safe.

Love: Wormwood is an herb that conquers anger, be it your own or that between people.

As a love charm, wormwood brings healthy, peaceful energy that can attract partners with similar energy.

Clearing: Wormwood clears excessive anger that can cloud your vision and stop you from seeing alternative solutions.

Healing: Clearing anger, promoting visions of alternate solutions, and connecting divine forces, wormwood can bring a deeper peace to your journey. It is also used to develop psychic powers.

YARROW

Healing
Yarrow is an herb whose energy is connected to the divine—listening to, getting guidance from, trusting in, and giving your problems over to a higher power.

Prosperity: Use yarrow when your financial issues are overwhelming and you see no way out. It can work to release those fears and allow you to be given the wisdom you need to create a better situation.

Protection: Yarrow protects you from self-sabotage by clearing the depression and melancholy that are triggering it.

Love: This is very effective to increase love and understanding between couples by clearing

the intense negative emotions that discord can generate. Yarrow also draws helpful friends and the attention of those you most want to talk to.

Clearing: Yarrow helps in finally releasing a long-standing depression by cleansing unhealthy fears and overwhelming sorrow and stopping self-negation.

Healing: Through its use in *I Ching* divination, yarrow connects you directly to divine wisdom. With the support of the divine your fears are replaced by courage, allowing the healing of emotional wounds and developing boundaries against the negativity from others.

YLANG-YLANG

Love
This essential oil is a wonderfully relaxing scent whose magic revolves around grounded and centered love.

Prosperity: Ylang-ylang can help calm the fears that can block prosperity's healthy presence in your life.

Protection: Use it to create a grounded and centered calm that helps you maintain balance in times of trauma that destroy your protective forces.

Love: Ylang-ylang creates sexual desire and promotes deepening love. It helps overcome fear and creates a relaxed attitude that increases confidence and warmth toward others.

Clearing: An aromatherapeutic antidepressant, it can relieve irritation, impatience, and anxiety.

Healing: Ylang-ylang is a wonderfully relaxing essence whose magic brings a sense of peace and a connection to a calm center.

WORKS REFERENCED AND SUGGESTED FURTHER READING

On Herbs and Oils

Beyerl, Paul. *The Master Book of Herbalism.* Blaine, WA: Phoenix Publishing, 1984.

Beyerl, Paul. *A Compendium of Herbal Magick.* Blaine, WA: Phoenix Publishing, 1998.

Cunningham, Scott. *Cunningham's Encyclopedia of Magical Herbs.* St. Paul, MN: Llewellyn Publications, 1996.

Grieve, Margaret. *A Modern Herbal.* 2 vols. Mineola, NY: Dover Publications, 1971. Also available online at *www.botanical.com.*

Worwood, Valerie Ann. *The Fragrant Mind: Aromatherapy for Personality, Mind, Mood, and Emotion.* Novato, CA: New World Library, 1996.

Yronwode, Catherine. *Hoodoo Herb and Root Magic: A Materia Magica of African-American Conjure.* Forestville, CA: Lucky Mojo Curio Company, 2002.

CRYSTAL AND STONE INDEX

This quick reference guide is to inspire the inclusion of crystals and stones in your spells. Whatever stones draw your attention while you are thinking of your spell are the ones that want in on the magic. There are more uses for stones than can be included in any one book. They give me new ideas about their magical purpose every time I bring them into my daily magic. Talk to your stones, explore their energy, and have fun on this journey!

AGATE (ALL TYPES)

Love, Healing
Overall, agate promotes a spiritual connection and an expanded perceptiveness in all situations. Including agate in your spell allows you to see and feel its outreaching effects.

Prosperity: Agate brings balance to abundance, helping it to anchor into your life. It has an analytical vibration that helps you understand all the options in front of you.

Protection: Agate will expand your perceptiveness in all situations.
Love: Agate promotes fidelity and loyalty in relationships.
Clearing: Agate brings an alignment to body, mind, and spirit, thus pushing out any discord or disharmony.
Healing: Agate realigns all the layers of the self, balancing yin and yang, and awakens inner wisdom and talent.

AMAZONITE

Protection, Clearing, Healing
Amazonite's main energy is soothing to your emotions and nerves and dispels negative energy.

Prosperity: Use amazonite in spells where you need to calm and soothe financial worries. It protects against unfair business practices. It is also great for luck, especially in risky investments.

Protection: Amazonite helps in protecting you from unwanted influence from any source.
Love: It calms emotions and helps connect people at the heart level, dispelling loneliness and returning happiness to marriages.
Clearing: Amazonite dispels negative energy and aggravation, smoothing your energy.
Healing: Its aligning and balancing energy is perfect for gentle healing spells.

AMBER

Prosperity, Protection, Healing

Amber is a stone of transformation; it brings order out of chaos, transmutes negative energy to positive, and transforms thoughts into tangible results.

Prosperity: Amber fills you with vital energy to give you the stamina and will to manifest through difficulty. It helps you find tangible actions to manifest your intent. It particularly draws investors.

Protection: Amber is very protective of children, shielding them from negativity and creating an ultimate sense of well-being and personal power.

Love: This stone stabilizes relationships through difficult times. It creates feelings of beauty inside and out.

Clearing: Amber dispels depression to bring joy and warmth.

Healing: Amber powers up your natural vitality and transforms negative energy and thoughts into positive. Amber connects the psychical body to divine forces.

AMETHYST

Protection, Love, Clearing, Healing

Spells cast with the added energy of amethyst are protected, balanced, and higher in vibration.

Prosperity: Use amethyst in business spells to help you clear influences to make shrewd business decisions. It clears self-doubt and greed, aligning you with the laws of Universal Abundance.

Protection: Amethyst protects against psychic attack and from being gaslighted into believing illusions. It protects against abuse.

Love: Amethyst transmutes negative influences into love. Use amethyst in spells when all parties need to see the higher purpose of a situation, to get someone to understand your point of view in a calm way, and to convince someone to take a chance on you.

Clearing: Just holding amethyst will help clear your aura and balance all levels of the self. It eases tension and energies that could disrupt your spell.

Healing: Meditating with amethyst before you cast your spell will bring a sense of calm contentedness. It connects you to divinity to cocreate your intention. Amethyst is perfect in spells for healing, by being soothing, calming, and tranquilizing in stressful situations.

AQUAMARINE

Protection, Clearing, Healing

The stone of courage, aquamarine helps to overcome fears that are preventing you from speaking your truth. Associated with the waters of the earth, it will sharpen your psychic senses.

Prosperity: Aquamarine connects you to the ebb and flow of the endless sea and sharpens your intuition to understand how to use its momentum. Use it in spells where you are speaking and teaching to clear fears, share your truth, and create a following.

Protection: Aquamarine is a stone of justice as it brings a natural balance to any situation. Use it in protection spells for stressful confrontations and to be able to negotiate with courage and clarity.

Love: Aquamarine helps soothe arguments and pushes everyone to find harmony together. Use it in spells for longevity in loving relationships.

Clearing: Aquamarine calms the mind, especially in overwhelming situations. It will bring closure to highly emotional situations.

Healing: Aquamarine promotes self-expression by clearing what is blocking it. Use it in spells to open your intuition and psychic senses.

AVENTURINE, GREEN

Prosperity, Clearing, Healing

This money stone is a powerful addition to any financial and success spells. It's known as the stone of opportunity because it brings optimism and an entrepreneurial spirit.

Prosperity: Use a piece of aventurine in every money and business spell to increase your optimism and entrepreneurial spirit.

Protection: Employ aventurine in protection spells to bring courage and the tenacity to burn through any energy that blocks you.

Love: Aventurine balances the male and female energies and helps you tap into your own wisdom.

Clearing: It activates and clears the old habits, fears, and inner sabotage that lie in the heart chakra. Keep an aventurine near you to shield your aura from the hooks of others.

Healing: Use it in spells that awaken your inner wisdom to help with making tough decisions. When you start working with this stone, be prepared to start assuming leadership roles.

BLOODSTONE

Prosperity, Protection, Healing

Known as the "stone of courage" and purification, bloodstone helps in any spell or intention by clearing negativity—including your own.

Prosperity: Use bloodstone in spells for respect and notoriety in your career or industry that can turn into good fortune and financial reward.

Protection: Bloodstones bring protection from negative, confusing, or abusive influences. Use bloodstone in any spell where turmoil and chaos are wreaking havoc. It helps in understanding the value in the current lesson so you can rebalance and clear.

Love: Use bloodstone in spells where you need protection in relationships that have become abusive in bullying or physical ways. It brings the courage needed to leave when the opportunity arrives.

Clearing: Use it in clearing spells to calm the mind, release confusion, and ground into the present moment. Bloodstone will promote clearing even if you are experiencing great anxiety.

Healing: Bloodstone boosts energy levels, builds stamina, and brings courage to any healing spell. Bloodstone will also help you understand the effect your spell will have on others.

CALCITE (ALL COLORS)

Prosperity, Clearing, Healing
Calcite is an amazing amplifier and cleanser of energy, making it an excellent stone to have on your altar when you are initializing a spell.

Prosperity: Calcite is an active stone that can be added to any spell to speed its growth.

Protection: Use calcite in protection spells that can be improved by the energy of discernment and analysis of the entire situation.

Love: Red calcite is used in spells to stimulate your will and passion.

Clearing: All calcite clears stagnant energy, thus boosting your overall energy.

Healing: Calcite can be used in spells that involve finding and actualizing your destiny; it is also good for revitalizing your own energy, especially when doing big spells.

CARNELIAN

Prosperity, Protection, Love, Healing
Any spell that increases or taps into the power of a woman is enhanced by carnelian. It grounds you into and empowers you with your present reality.

Prosperity: Use in career-building and wealth-building spells to pull in hidden and unexpected resources.

Protection: Carnelian protects from envy, fear, and rage. Use this in spells to increase courage, build better personal boundaries, and have the will to enforce them.

Love: It is also a good choice for spells that affect the energy in the lower chakras: creation, sexuality, life force, and will.

Clearing: Use carnelian in spells that clear blocks to creativity. It is also useful when a fear of failure is preventing you from even starting.

Healing: Use carnelian in spells to restore lost motivation and vitality. It also brings stability to feminine goddess energy, so it can empower spells of nurturing, creation, and compassion.

CITRINE

Prosperity
Known as the merchant's stone, citrine can be added to your money spells to help you to gain, maintain, and protect your wealth.

Prosperity: Citrine increases your overall energy and strengthens the part of your will that brings about the manifestation of your dreams. Add this to any spells for money, success, career, and fame.

Protection: Citrine is very useful in protection spells; it does not hold or accumulate negative energies, but instead dissipates and transmutes them. It will keep your protection spells energized.

Love: Citrine is also good for soothing group or family problems that are caused by a clash of wills.

Clearing: Citrine works to increase your personal power, creativity, and intelligence by bringing clarity of thought, mental focus, and endurance.

Healing: By using citrine in your spells, you connect to your higher self and bring the love and support of the universe to you.

EMERALD

Protection, Love, Healing
A powerful love stone, emerald is known as the stone of successful love.

Prosperity: Use emerald in spells to promote understanding in a business partnership. It will also bring a deeper understanding and wisdom in any situation.

Protection: Emerald protects from misfortune and misunderstandings.

Love: Use emerald in spells for domestic bliss, happy marriages, partnerships, and friendship. It brings a higher understanding of love as well as patience and positive actions.

Clearing: Emerald draws in joy and positivity, displacing disruptive and chaotic energies.

Healing: Use emerald in spells to increase psychic abilities or that need an open intuition.

FLUORITE

Protection, Clearing, Healing
The structured energy of fluorite affects the body, mind, and spirit, bringing clarity to every level of the self.

Prosperity: Use fluorite in spells where the chaos around you is causing financial stress.

Protection: Use fluorite in protection spells when life feels chaotic and you need protection, or when you are in crisis in any way.

Love: Use it in love spells when you are unsure of the other party's interest.

Clearing: It helps one to see the truth and reality that were hidden under the confusion.

Healing: Fluorite is very soothing to the spirit, calming and clearing an agitated energy field. It will also help you pick one idea out of the many and focus on it. Fluorite is also a wonderful stone to have in a classroom to bring a mental order to all the information the student is absorbing.

GARNET

Protection, Love

Garnet is a reenergizing stone that promotes health, passion, protection, and a balanced energy field.

Prosperity: Garnet strengthens survival instincts. Use it in money spells where you need courage, hope, and strength of character to get through a crisis.

Protection: Add garnet to protective spells to warn of danger.

Love: Use garnet in spells to inspire love and balance sexual energy.

Clearing: Garnet pulls discordant and negative energy from your chakras and replaces it with balanced energy.

Healing: Use garnet in spells to increase and balance your vital energy.

HEMATITE

Protection, Clearing

Hematite's grounding and protective vibration brings balance to all levels of the self. It keeps you in your body while you explore high-vibration mental and spiritual information.

Prosperity: Use hematite in spells where you have limited your personal power or ability to achieve. It opens you up to more ideas and possibilities.

Protection: Add it to spells where you are overcoming fears that hold you back and keep you timid. Hematite will power up your courage and protect you while you are finding your voice.

Love: Use hematite in spells where you are finding the confidence to pursue your love interest.

Clearing: Hematite will clear negative intentions from others and prevent them from reattaching to your energy field.

Healing: Hematite brings mental clarity to cut through excess thoughts and focus on one idea at a time. Hematite is also good for spells to support breaking addictions.

JADE

Prosperity, Protection, Healing
Wisdom, purity, and tranquility are the attributes of jade that have been held sacred for 6,000 years.

Prosperity: The presence of jade in any spell brings overall blessings. It helps you find your life's purpose and be your own authentic self.

Protection: Use jade in protection spells for long life, good health, and peaceful endings. It wards off spiritual attacks.

Love: Use it in love spells to keep from losing your identity to the relationship you are chasing.

Clearing: Jade calms the mind in the middle of a storm and brings blessing to every area of your life.

Healing: Use jade in spells to find and fulfill your destiny as it awakens your true self.

JASPER

Protection, Healing
Jasper comes in many varieties and is known for the pictures found within the stones. It is called the supreme nurturer, as all types of jasper bring support and tranquility in times of stress.

Prosperity: Add jasper to your prosperity spells when your energy is being drained by constant financial stress. It will bring stability and tranquility and reenergize your vital body.

Protection: Use jasper in spells to protect and ground the energy in your physical body.

Love: Employ it in lust spells to prolong sexual pleasure.

Clearing: Use jasper in spells where you need emotional stability to get through clearing addictions and bad habits.

Healing: Applied in spells for confidence, jasper will power up your determination and courage to act assertively when needed.

JET

Protection, Clearing, Healing
This deep-black stone is actually petrified wood and one of the primary stones of protection, making it a welcome addition to any spell of that nature.

Prosperity: Jet is helpful in spells that stabilize and protect your finances, both personal and business. It also brings mastery with manifesting your intent and showing its full potential.

Protection: Use jet in spells to protect against violence, to keep from falling prey to darker forces, and as protection in shamanic journeys. It empowers your energetic fields and creates a force of protection around you.

Love: Jet helps you take control of your life, making it useful in spells where you are taking back power in unhealthy relationships.

Clearing: Jet will cleanse the mind of fearful thoughts, help dispel depression, and strengthen the aura by keeping it clear and transmuting negative energy into something usable.

Healing: Jet helps open your psychic centers and assists you on your quest for spiritual enlightenment. It's protective and grounding and surrounds you with the elements, safeguarding your spirit on the journey.

LABRADORITE

Protection, Healing

Known as the stone of destiny, labradorite puts us in touch with our higher self and higher purpose.

Prosperity: This stone is also good for translating intuition into practical knowledge that can be used in a manifestation spell.

Protection: Labradorite protects your aura from invasive, unwanted energy and prevents energy leaks or hooks from others.

Love: Use it in spells to bring out the best in people and temper the negative side of the personality.

Clearing: It will strengthen and protect your aura from the hooks, drains, and drama of others. Ultimately, this stone brings a higher awareness of who you are and how you affect the world.

Healing: Use it in spells to help you rise above any self-imposed limitations to reach for your destiny. When you use this stone, all your natural psychic gifts will awaken and grow, and access to the Akashic records will be easier to attain.

LAPIS

Protection, Clearing, Healing

Lapis opens the third eye and enhances all types of psychic abilities. It is known as the stone of truth, and it enhances all mental activity and discernment.

Prosperity: Use lapis in spells to understand what next steps in prosperity and success are best. It helps you internalize all the wisdom you have gained through life's lessons.

Protection: Lapis brings out the truth in any situation and protects your mental processes.

Love: Use lapis in relationship spells where the expression of emotions is needed to bring a conflict to closure. It will also bring a deeper understanding of the universal truth of a situation.

Clearing: Employ it in spells to bring out truth and honesty to bring a deeper inner wisdom.

Healing: In spells that enhance spiritual growth, dream work, vision work, it helps you find your own inner truth, empowering the expression of your opinions and emotions.

LEPIDOLITE

Clearing, Healing

Known as the stone of transition, lepidolite brings a cosmic awareness of life's purpose. It deflects electromagnetic pollution, spirit attachments, and the overwhelming emotions from others.

Prosperity: Use lepidolite in prosperity spells that need focused, quick decision-making free of distractions.

Protection: Use it in protection spells where you are preventing the influence of others.

Love: Apply lepidolite in love spells to prevent being obsessive in your pursuit or to protect you from the obsession of others.

Clearing: Lepidolite is helpful in spells that support clearing addictions and obsessions.

Healing: Lepidolite assists in finding a mental and emotional balance in the middle of distractions. It helps to focus on what is for your highest good.

LODESTONE (MAGNETITE)

Prosperity, Protection, Love, Clearing

This is a magnetic stone that has positive-negative poles. It attracts what you most desire.

Prosperity: Use a lodestone with magnetic sand in money draw spells.

Protection: Lodestone is very grounding and can be used in protection spells to power your protective field.

Love: Pair lodestones in spells where you are attracting a specific person.

Clearing: A lodestone can be used in clearing spells to pull disruptive energy off of you and ground it into the earth.

Healing: Lodestones can balance your male and female polarities. Its grounding energy aids in psychic abilities, meditation, and visualization.

MOONSTONE

Love, Clearing, Healing

Moonstone brings you closer to the female aspect of divinity and helps you flow with what the creatrix has in store for you.

Prosperity: Moonstone is a powerful tool for embodying the creative energies of the universe to use them in manifesting your intention.

Protection: Use moonstone in a protection spell to help you alleviate turmoil-induced stress. It's also used in travel spells, as it brings protection and patience.

Love: Use it in love spells to help you accept the nurturing qualities of love. It is excellent in spells that awaken eroticism and lusty desires.

Clearing: Moonstone is excellent in spells to help you let go of limiting emotional patterns due to trauma. It clears stress and emotional overload.

Healing: It helps a person see and maintain their destiny, increases intuition and insight, and enhances perception and discernment. Use

moonstone in spells to bring a balancing, introspective, reflective, and lunar energy. Moonstone allows you to see endings as new beginnings.

OBSIDIAN, BLACK

Protection, Clearing, Healing

Obsidian's energy is boundless and increases the speed of your magic. Its energy is mirrorlike, showing you the shadow parts of the self and helping you understand their purpose in your life.

Prosperity: Obsidian works well in spells that uncover the blocks to your prosperity and how you manifested them.

Protection: Add obsidian to protective spells to create a force field against negative energies.

It helps you ground and reenergize to face the negative energies that are affecting you.

Love: Use it in spells that help you understand your part in what is going wrong in your relationships.

Clearing: Obsidian will draw out all negative energies whether they are yours or from an attack.

Healing: When applied in spells for spiritual growth, obsidian will help you understand your fears and blocks, allowing the spells to clear what is stopping you from connecting with your life's purpose.

OPAL

Love, Healing

Opal is a karmic stone that teaches you what you send out comes back to you. It collects the energy that you are sending out and intensifies it in your own life.

Prosperity: Use opal in prosperity spells to enhance your self-worth and help you see your full potential.

Protection: Opal in protection spells will make you unnoticeable or invisible.

Love: Employ opal in love spells to heighten passion and desire. Opal is seductive and releases sexual inhibitions.

Clearing: Use this stone in spells where you need to clear emotions that are stuck in the past.

Healing: Opal strengthens the will to live, making it a powerful addition to your healing spells. Additionally, opal aligns you to your spiritual purpose and soothes your fears around actualizing that. Opal also enhances psychic abilities.

PETRIFIED WOOD

Protection, Healing

Petrified wood is grounding and transformative in its energy. It brings patience for your spiritual evolution and helps you stay true to your path.

Prosperity: Use petrified wood in financial spells for your money to take root in your life and create security. Petrified wood represents a solid foundation for your intention for a candle spell to launch from. It works well for good-fortune spells.

Protection: Apply it in protection spells where you are creating an impenetrable fortress with a strong foundation.

Love: In happy marriage/partnership spells petrified wood supports a solid foundation. Use it in relationship spells to calm the fears that come from an insecure foundation.

Clearing: Use it in spells when you feel stuck or frozen in a specific way of being and thinking.

Healing: Petrified wood keeps you connected with the energies of the earth. In spells for personal transformation it helps you to stay true to the course.

QUARTZ CRYSTAL

Prosperity, Protection, Love, Clearing, Healing

Quartz crystal is the most common stone on the planet, and it's also the most powerful healing and energy stone on the planet. It manages your energy in many ways: storing it, amplifying it, directing it, and regulating it. It quickens your magic and is programmable for any spell you are casting.

Prosperity: Quartz will amplify your prosperity spell and accelerate its manifestation.

Protection: Use quartz to set up a powerful protection grid in coordination with your candle spell.

Love: Quartz works in love spells to raise the vibration of your intent to the highest quality and for your highest good.

Clearing: Use it in clearing spells to pull out dissonant energy and heal your spirit and energy.

Healing: The ultimate healing stone, quartz functions in spells to awaken deep and ancient knowledge.

ROSE QUARTZ

Love, Healing

Rose quartz is the stone of unconditional love. It raises the vibration of all emotions to a healing and loving height, exemplifying the true essence of love.

Prosperity: Rose quartz can be used in spells where finances are dependent on another person.

Protection: Use it in protection spells where your emotions are at risk. Rose quartz will draw off negative energy and set up a vibration of peace and love.

Love: The ultimate love stone, use rose quartz in all love and relationship spells.

Clearing: Rose quartz helps clear trauma and crisis, gently moving your heart chakra and emotions back to a healthy balance. Rose quartz will clear fears and resentments and replace them with a divine loving energy.

Healing: Use rose quartz in healing spells that need the divine feminine energy of compassion and peace. Rose quartz brings tender vibrations of nourishment and comfort as it speaks directly to the heart chakra to dissolve emotional wounds.

SELENITE

Prosperity, Protection, Love, Clearing, Healing

Named after the moon goddess Selene, selenite has an ethereal vibration and brings pure, healing white light into all of your magical spells.

Prosperity: Selenite is used in prosperity, success, and career spells to raise the vibration to a higher purpose and speed manifestation.

Protection: Use selenite in your protection spells to create a protective grid and shield.

Love: In love spells, selenite will bring a calm confidence. It is also helpful in connecting to people you knew in a past life.

Clearing: Selenite is used in healing work to draw out negative energies and rebalance you. It will help in detaching spiritual attachments and clearing hooks that are draining your energy.

Healing: Use it in all healing spells to open your psychic connection to divine energies and bring healing vibrations to all that you do.

SERPENTINE

Healing

Serpentine is a stone that opens up new mental pathways and psychic abilities.

Prosperity: Use serpentine in prosperity spells to bring a feeling of control over your circum-

stances. It supports the process of manifestation.

Protection: It is effective for protection spells where you are exploring other realms and past lives.

Love: Use serpentine in spells where you are looking to understand your spiritual connection with another.

Clearing: Add serpentine to any cleansing spells.

Healing: Use it in spells where you are opening up your psychic abilities and connection to spirit. When healing and aligning your chakras, serpentine can help you alter your energy to a new level and path.

SNOWFLAKE OBSIDIAN

Protection

This stone helps in recognizing and repatterning negative and self-destructive thoughts, thus supporting making the best out of a bad situation. This is particularly important when you are casting spells during times of crisis to remain clear and focused.

Prosperity: Use snowflake obsidian in prosperity spells to see your way through the crisis at hand.

Protection: In protection spells it will bring the courage, persistence, and hope needed to break any self-destructive pattern you are in. When protecting from outside influences, use snowflake obsidian not only to stop negative energy from entering the aura but also to break the hex and return it to its sender. Placed by the door, it stops unwanted guests from entering your home.

Love: Use snowflake obsidian in love spells where you are looking for a spiritual connection with others and to open new paths for love to enter your life.

Clearing: Carry this with you to clear your mind of obsessive thought and ground yourself in truth and reality.

Healing: This stone will help with meditation, bringing purity and balance to all levels of the self.

SODALITE

Clearing, Healing

Use sodalite in spells that involve unlocking your creativity, uncovering the truth, opening your throat chakra, and increasing your psychic abilities.

Prosperity: Sodalite is good in success and prosperity spells when you need introspection on what is working and what is not.

Protection: Use sodalite as a truth-seeking stone in protection spells.

Love: Add sodalite in spells where you are promoting fellowship, solidarity, and commonality of a goal for a group. Use it in relationship spells to enhance truthfulness and verbalize authentic feelings.

Clearing: Use sodalite in spells that clear out confusing information and bring out the truth of the situation.

Healing: The magical use of sodalite helps you process and analyze the intuitive and psychic impressions you receive during your ritual and intention work, transforming emotional confusion into a rational mental process.

SUNSTONE

Prosperity, Healing

Sunstone brings joy, inspiration, and a thirst for life. It illuminates the darker parts of your life and fills them with warmth and benevolence.

Prosperity: Use sunstone in spells where you are looking for blessings and good fortune in your finances and career as it has a very abundant and independent energy.

Protection: Apply sunstone in protection spells where your energy is being drained.

Love: Sunstone supports spells where you are opening to love and where it already exists in your life.

Clearing: Use sunstone in spells where you are clearing the hooks and drains from others. Sunstone will clear depression and dark moods.

Healing: Sunstone brings optimism and hope, making it an excellent addition to spells where you are building confidence and finding your self-worth.

TIGEREYE

Healing

Tigereye helps you intuitively know when to take action and how. This is extremely helpful in spellwork for knowing when to gather more energy and when to release it.

Prosperity: Use this stone in prosperity spells when the moment of action is critical, such as for gambling, investments, bidding, loans, and sales.

Protection: Employ tigereye in protection spells to see where the negative energy is coming from. It protects from ill wishes and curses.

Love: Use it in love spells where you are finding your courage and self-esteem to attract someone that respects you.

Clearing: In spells it will clear out the confusion that comes from too much or untrustworthy information.

Healing: Tigereye can also help you balance your extremes and find a middle or common ground in any situation, including bringing an emotional balance, making your spell more targeted and effective. It can soothe your vibrations and settle internal turmoil.

TOURMALINE, BLACK

Protection, Clearing

This is one of the most powerful stones to protect you from the negative energy sent to you from humans, spirits, and demons.

Prosperity: Use black tourmaline in prosperity spells to protect your good fortune from the envy and negative wishes of others.

Protection: Black tourmaline can act as a shield in protection spells to clear out and ward off hexes, curses, and evil eyes sent your way.

It will also protect you from negative spirits attaching to or affecting you.

Love: Use black tourmaline in clearing and breaking love spells that have gone bad.

Clearing: Employ black tourmaline to clear negative energy out of your aura and spirit.

It also is known to clear electromagnetic overload.

Healing: Black tourmaline is a good addition to all healing spells for body, spirit, and mind.

TURQUOISE

Prosperity, Protection, Love, Clearing, Healing
Turquoise is said to marry heaven and earth, bringing your visions to fruition and helping you to ground while maintaining a strong connection to the spiritual realm.

Prosperity: Add turquoise to your spell to bring it into perfect alignment with the forces of the universe.

Protection: Turquoise is good in spells to protect property and against accidents.

Love: Use turquoise in spells to empower those who are shy by helping them realize they have something important to share.

Clearing: Apply turquoise in spells that break the hold of illusion and show you the truth.

Healing: Turquoise strengthens and aligns all the chakras and all the elements, making it perfect for spiritual healing spells. It helps you understand the wisdom that culminates from all of life's experiences.

OTHER SOURCES FOR CRYSTAL MEANINGS

Judy Hall. *The Crystal Bible*. Iola, WI: Krause Publications, 2003.

Melody. *Love Is in the Earth: A Kaleidoscope of Crystals*. Wheat Ridge, CO: Earth-Love Publishing House, 1995.

Simmons, Robert, and Naisha Ahsian. *The Book of Stones: Who They Are and What They Teach*. East Montpelier, VT: Heaven & Earth Publishing, 2005.

Crystal Metaphysical Encyclopedia, *crystalvaults.com*

TAROT INDEX

0 FOOL

Beginning a journey or new part of your life. The truth of a situation will be revealed as the Fool does not know how to lie.

Prosperity: Use in spells where a new path of prosperity or material gain is needed.

Protection: Use to reveal the truth of a situation and get tangible proof.

Love: Use in spells to renew the fun in a relationship and fall in love all over again.

Clearing: Use to leave behind what no longer works and embrace the unknown.

Healing: Use in spells where the innocence and belief of your inner child are needed.

1 MAGICIAN

Mastery over a situation or subject. Enhanced creativity and use of all forces of creation.

Prosperity: Use in spells to gain mastery over your financial situation through leveraging all of your resources both at hand and hidden. Great for artists that are trying to monetize their works.

Protection: Use this to add personal control over a dangerous situation.

Love: Unblock and rethink habits or energies that keep you from forming a new relationship or deepening an existing one.

Clearing: Great for clearing blocks in pursuit of mastery of a skill.

Healing: This card can bring in all elements and hidden resources to assist in the healing process.

2 HIGH PRIESTESS

Another great card to uncover the truth of a situation, use this card for spells that include increasing your psychic intuition or empowering your womanly wiles.

Prosperity: Great for women in business to clear inequality or unjust actions that prevent professional growth.

Protection: Used to reveal whose energy may be causing you harm.

Love: Use in love spells to draw in the powers of feminine attraction and persuasion.

Clearing: Good to clear away lies and illusion to reveal the truth in a situation.

Healing: Use in spells to increase your intuition and arcane arts.

3 EMPRESS

This is perfect for fertility spells, specifically for becoming pregnant. Also use this card when you need growth in any situation. Great addition when you are looking for a new advisor—helps balance the Hierophant.

Prosperity: Good for all fertility spells, specifically pregnancy. Can be directed to bring abundance and wisdom to an expanding situation.

Protection: Use to protect children and pregnancies.

Love: Use to strengthen the bond between mother and child or in love spells to add nurturing energy.

Clearing: Use after a clearing spell to invite abundance into your life.

Healing: Use to invite growth after healing from trauma.

4 EMPEROR

When you need unchallenged power and authority in a situation. This card represents the merciful ruler, so in spells, it can balance your inner power. This is also a good card to use when you are building something (like an empire).

Prosperity: Good for personal empire building or increased fertility for those with a penis.

Protection: Use for unbending authority over your protection.

Love: Use to build a balanced relationship.

Clearing: Use to take authority over spirits or energies that may have their hooks in you and clear them from your life.

Healing: Use to take authority over your own healing. The Emperor will help you find your inner empowerment and overcome fears that keep you timid.

5 HIEROPHANT

The Hierophant is the keeper of traditions and the great teacher. Use this card if you need to

find a teacher/advisor or bring logic and stability to a situation.

Prosperity: Employers can use this card in spells to attract, hire, and retain talented staff. Can also be used to find advisory services to expand or stabilize business. Employees can use this card in spells to find a workplace whose culture and traditions match their energy.

Protection: Use this card to attract allies to aid in your defense and bring wise advice against advisories.

Love: Use this card to attract wise and long-term friends with a wealth of experience that is different from your own.

Clearing: Use this card to critically think about what needs to be cleared from your life.

Healing: Use this card to expand your spiritual wisdom and find a teacher to help this growth.

6 LOVERS

The Lovers is more about choice than romance. Use this card if you are in an uncertain love situation to make a decision. Use in spells where you suspect infidelity to force a decision from the other party. Use in marriage spells to strengthen the bond between the couple and celebrate surviving the trials and challenges of life.

Prosperity: Use this card in spells to stabilize professional relationships and partnerships.

Protection: Use this card to uncover unknowingly toxic relationships and confront toxic traits in a process of cutting ties or healing a relationship.

Love: Use this card to rekindle long-term relationships that may have become stagnant.

Clearing: Use this card in reverse to sever ties with long-term relationships. Warning, employing the card this way will permanently cut these links and could also end associated relationships—do not use this method on a whim.

Healing: Use this card in healing long-term relationships that may have become frayed, whether that be with lovers, friends, or family. Apply in spells where you have a difficult decision to make.

7 CHARIOT

Use to blast through blocks and open the road to your success. Add this to your spell if you want to move fast, but be aware that you may lose control of the speed. A great addition if you are looking to gain an alliance from your opposites.

Prosperity: This is your fast cash card, but beware of it going out as fast as it comes in.

Best for influxes of cash for emergency situations like a car repair or medical bill.

Protection: Turns enemies into allies, but this move comes with a considerable amount of risk, although it may also have a great payoff.

Love: Use this card for a drastic change in your relationship, best as a final change or test. The new change will lead to either reconciliation or separation.

Clearing: Powerfully blast through entrenched blocks in your life.

Healing: This is the equivalent of putting a Band-Aid on a cut that needs stitches: it will help stem the bleeding but won't fix the root cause.

---

8 STRENGTH

This card is used for courage and faith and to tap into the inner reserves of your power. When all feels lost, use this card in your spell.

Prosperity: Find your inner strength to make large or energetically draining economic decisions to tap into your hidden reserves.

Protection: Find your inner power to confront an uncomfortable situation.

Love: Use this to muster courage to set and follow boundaries with relationships you want to maintain in your life.

Clearing: Use this to have the courage to let go of and release energy that may have been comforting or served you in some way, but no longer has a place in your life.

Healing: Use this card to face unspoken and uncovered traumas that you are ready to heal from. It can bring a calm perspective when you are filled with panic.

---

9 HERMIT

Use the Hermit to call an advisor to you. Also this card can serve when you are looking for answers to seemingly insurmountable problems or issues that keep cropping up. It can be helpful to uncover the truth of any situation.

Prosperity: Use this card in spells to gain the confidence of your boss. This is also useful in spells where you are breaking an unhealthy financial cycle in your life and learning a new way to be.

Protection: Use this card in spells to call allies that are best equipped to prevent repeated attacks. The Hermit can help in constructing the language for legal documents, briefs, and arguments in your party's favor.

Love: This card is great to explore your relationship with yourself and your own ego. It can help answer questions requiring deep thought.

Clearing: This card will act as your Marie Kondo clearing master. When you are faced with seemingly insurmountable energies that do not "spark joy," use this card as an assistant to get organized, thank the energy for its time, and let it go.

Healing: This card will help heal the root cause of an issue. Damage or traumas that continually reoccur are caused by a root problem or repeated action which this card will help identify.

10 WHEEL OF FORTUNE

Use this to turn luck in your direction, but if it's already on your side, it could turn it away from you instead. This is also a card to uncover your destiny so you may more easily follow it.

Prosperity: Use this if economics finds you in a downturn to switch your position to an upturn.
Protection: Use this card to reverse your position with your attackers, and the negative energies they send you will be turned on them.
Love: Use this card to change emotions within a relationship, especially if they are currently sour.
Clearing: Use this card to reverse the flow of energy, in this case from into your life to out of your life.
Healing: Use this card in spells where you need to understand the ebb and flow of your life.

11 JUSTICE

In legal matters this card will help justice to be in your favor.

Prosperity: Use for financial lawsuits.
Protection: Works in gaining favor for a restraining order or any other protection orders.
Love: Use in making lasting marriage licenses or smooth adoptions.
Clearing: Use in settling or dismissing lawsuits.
Healing: Supports recovering from a painful or lengthy legal battle.

12 HANGED MAN

This is a card for learning the wisdom that resides deep within. It also helps you see through the illusion of lies. This is a card to bring mastery through experience in situations of leadership and wisdom.

Prosperity: Use this card to discover and develop leadership skills at work as a boss or an employee looking for a promotion.
Protection: Investigate truth and your personal truth in a negative situation.
Love: A card of self-exploration to understand the truths about yourself and how they affect your relationships. This is also excellent with setting boundaries.
Clearing: When healing from past traumas, this card is great at severing the links in time that are causing illness and discomfort.
Healing: Use this card to discard the pieces of yourself that no longer serve you and clear self-contained negative energies.

13 DEATH

This is the card of big change! Total transformation and endings come from this energy. Use this card if you want to end something, but be very, very specific. It's also a good card to help let go of the past.

Prosperity: Use this card to end specific business ventures or for firings of employees, customers, or bosses. Be *hyper*specific about your targeted break.

Protection: Surgically break negative bonds.

Love: Use to break a relationship with a person. Make sure you name them in your spell or it could bring down any supportive networks.

Clearing: When used to permanently and severely sever ties, like a forest after a fire, this card will leave fertile ground for anything to grow—whether it be weeds or flowers.

Healing: If this card comes up in a reading, use the card from the reading to start your healing journey. It is a sign to let go of what is hurting you.

14 TEMPERANCE

Use this card to bring balance to any situation, tempering two opposites to create a strong and balanced center point. This is also a card for situations that seem hopeless, as there is always a new answer to be crafted from the raw materials of the problem at hand.

Prosperity: Create a balanced flow of work with a healthy return on investment. You can also use this card to calm and balance any unsustainable growth or spiraling shrinkage.

Protection: Use this to establish a safe situation, curb random attacks, and bring a sense of order.

Love: Use this to balance the power dynamics in a relationship, between business partners, friends, or lovers. It is great for creating stable communication about needs and boundaries.

Clearing: This is used to break down everything to its nearest bones or roots.

Healing: This is the card to rebuild and heal after a complete base-level clearing.

15 DEVIL

Use this card in a spell to encourage greed, lust, and materialism. You can also use it in a reversed position to break obsessions and bring a new direction in life. This is very helpful for spells to break the hold of a past lover.

Prosperity: This is a card that serves capitalism, inviting materialism and greed. Use this card in the reverse to banish obsessive energy from your business practices.

Protection: This card is good for casting protections against stalker energy.

Love: This card is good for breaking connections with a past lover.

Clearing: Use this card in reverse to banish habits, people, and places that feed your internal saboteur.

Healing: Use this card as a garbage disposal for devilish habits in yourself and around your energy.

16 TOWER

Use reversed to limit the amount of turmoil in your life. Use in the upright position if you need to make a great change and want to shake your or someone else's foundation to the core. The Tower can be used to create trouble in someone else's life.

Prosperity: This card reverses misfortunes in revenue or in situations of continued loss.

Protection: At times when you suspect you are under psychic attack, use this card in reverse to return curses to the sender.

Love: Use this card to drastically shake up your relationships. In reverse it will stop unfounded conflict.

Clearing: Use this card in a laser focus to clear out a stuck situation. In reverse it can be used to quickly banish your target to the shadow realm.

Healing: Use in the reversed position to stop turmoil so you can see and heal the fears, blocks, or beliefs that are creating chaos.

17 STAR

When things seem hopeless and desperate, use this card to bring hope, faith, and the connection to the divine. This is another card to use to bring new prospects into the picture.

Prosperity: Use this card to find your way out of a tricky situation. This card will bring hope and a new perspective to drastic financial situations. Use to create an amicable resolution in any work situation or to be the star candidate when looking for a job.

Protection: Use this with other protection cards to add positive energy in a resolution that works in your favor.

Love: Use with other cards to kindle new relationships and love.

Clearing: Use to invite positive energies to occupy the space left by a clearing.

Healing: Use to bring hope, positive energy, and stamina to healing, especially for physical illness.

18 MOON

Uncovers lies that have been hidden by emotion and suspect behavior. Also useful in heightening your intuition in a matter, to know instinctively where the truth resides.

Prosperity: Clear emotional blocks to grow your business. Use this card to get out of your own way and refocus on goals.

Protection: Increase your awareness to locate the source of a threat.

Love: Bring intuition into disagreements, particularly between lovers.

Clearing: Great for clearing emotional baggage that may be clouding a healing process.

Healing: Use to bring feminine energies into the healing process, particularly around emotional damage caused by lies. Use to empower your intuition and grow your psychic skills.

19 SUN

Success! Use this card to bring success and joy to any situation. This is a victory card to be brought to bear in any spell where you need to overcome or burn through an obstacle. Remember, the Sun overrides everything.

Prosperity: Use this card to close deals, complete projects, and meet financial goals in abundance.

Protection: The heat from the card is great for creating barriers of transformative energy.

Love: Use this card to help yourself be heard in a relationship, whether with your boss, peers, or a lover. Be careful, though: the sun trumps everything so you must be open to listen while your opinion shines through. Can also be directed to bring fun and joy into your relationships.

Clearing: The brightness of this card vaporizes energy like a UV disinfecting light. Use this card to burn away stubborn, clingy energies.

Healing: Use this card to clear blocks you may encounter on your healing journey and add a gentle glowing light to your growth.

20 JUDGMENT

Use this card to gain your awaited rewards for your efforts. This card also helps you let go of and atone for your past.

Prosperity: Use this card to correct and resolve past business mistakes that may be holding you back.

Protection: Use this card to identify threats from your past you wish to protect against.

Love: Use this card with a partner to apologize for mistakes of the past and move to a new beginning. Can also be used to achieve a final emotional release on past relationships.

Clearing: Use this card to forgive yourself and unpack past trauma to release it. Good for uncovering and handling past family or generational traumas.

Healing: Use this card to transition into a new beginning after your healing process.

---

21 WORLD

Use this card when you are unsure of what your next step will be. This is also a card to turn to in gentle endings—versus the extreme endings of the Death card. It will also help make a change of location.

Prosperity: Use this card to help answer questions of how to take the next steps in your professional life or business. Also use this card when you are moving to ensure your new location will be a blessing.

Protection: Use this card when you are looking for a new space to ensure that that space is safe for you.

Love: Use this card to determine or strengthen next steps with your partner, whether that is by moving in together or getting married.

Clearing: Use this as a gentle cleanser, to break ties with a situation or person whom you wish the best but who no longer fits into your life.

Healing: Use this card to actualize your own personal power.

PENTACLES

The pentacles are a suit geared at financial situations, so they will work best for you in such situations. This does not mean that you cannot use these cards in other ways, but spells connected with material possessions, finances, and business will see the best results.

Ace of Pentacles

Use to bring new opportunities for financial increase like a new job, luck, or new business venture. Also brings new physical pleasure. Helps ground and center you in your new opportunity into your current life.

Prosperity: This card shines in financial situations, which brings luck and unplanned windfalls to business.

Protection: Use this to protect your new opportunities while you are making decisions or keep you from inadvertently falling victim to scams while exploring.

Love: This card can been used in matters of sex. Whether you're trying something new or looking to enhance your current practices, this card will amplify your process.

Clearing: Use this card to help ground you in your clearing process and remain focused on your target.

Healing: Use this card to ground yourself, especially if you are healing inner issues related to money, finances, and material possessions.

King of Pentacles

This card represents a good businessperson who can create fortunes from new ideas. He is kind and loyal and can separate business from pleasure. Most likely he is a leader in his field and good with money. You can also use this card to help close real estate deals in your direction or if you need a new business idea.

Prosperity: This card is good for situations needing creativity or anything to do with real estate sales or materialistic success. As a King this card is particularly powerful for those who work in male energies.

Protection: This is great when drafting legal documents for a business or employee contracts.

Love: This card is best utilized by those with masculine energies to find a stable business partner.

Clearing: Pentacles is a suit connected with the five elements, including spirit, and its cards are great for use in elemental clearings. In reverse the King will also banish greedy tendencies that may standing in the way of your financial growth.

Healing: This card is good in healing situations of systematic financial misstep, whether it be getting into the wrong job and needing to find a new one or recovering from employee theft. This card will help heal that situation.

Queen of Pentacles

This card represents a down-to-earth woman who has an excellent business sense. She loves nature and beautiful things and is very committed to her family. This card can also be used for success in business deals, taking control of your work situation, or sticking to a health/diet plan. Combined with the Empress, it promotes fertility.

Prosperity: This card is great for solidifying good business practices and routines. Whereas the King of Pentacles represents more of a corporate business energy, the Queen symbolizes local family and community businesses.

Protection: This card is great for protecting family or generational finances.

Love: This card is good for using the elements to anchor familial love. Employ this card with the Empress to promote fertility.

Clearing: Use this card to clear blockages in the family to generational and community growth.

Healing: Use this card to commit to new health regimes.

Knight of Pentacles

This card represents a teen or young adult who loves the finer things in life. He can be secretive, but it is just his need for solitude. Use this card when you need your business venture to move to the next level or to transform a seemingly lost venture into a moneymaker.

Prosperity: This card is transformative, turning negative times into prosperous ones.

Protection: Use the Knight of Pentacles to protect your business ideas or ventures when you are taking risks to start or expand your business or invest money. This is good for the protection of adolescents during their explorative years.

Love: This card is great for transforming an interpersonal conflict into a moment of growth and improvement in the relationship.

Clearing: This card can help create a solitary space for meditative clearing.

Healing: The reverse of this card can be used to establish a healthy work balance and develop good habits.

Page of Pentacles

This court card represents a child who likes to make things with dirt, sand, mud, or anything from nature. She is very industrious and not afraid to work for her money. If not used to represent a person, it can be used to represent getting a new idea or a message about a career/job move or from a loved one far away.

Prosperity: This card is about hard work and success through toil and trial. Use it to bring new or increased work and responsibilities into your life.

Protection: This card will aid in building long-term protective practices and making permanent moves into a safer space.

Love: This card is great for relationship building, particularly for new relationships that are maturing.

Clearing: Use this card in reverse to clear away opportunities and responsibilities that you can no longer manage.

Healing: Use this as an aid in healing deep trauma, to find the will to continue the hard but right path forward.

10 of Pentacles

This card represents financial security that will last a lifetime and beyond. Use this card to support building your empire, creating a stable family life, and attaining real property.

Prosperity: Use this card to create long-term financial stability. It's not necessarily about becoming the next multibillionaire, but rather about securing your financial future after retirement and property in your name for you and your children.

Protection: This card will protect your long-term investments and generational wealth.

Love: This card is about building long-term relationships. Deepen a connection with a soul mate to last a lifetime.

Clearing: This card will help clear financial instability from your home or office.

Healing: Use to manifest long-term health for your financial energy and to heal family legacies around money.

9 of Pentacles

This card represents having the financial stability to enjoy luxury. Use it if you need a windfall of cash, but be aware this also means you will be spending it alone. If solace is what you are looking for, this is what you will get.

Prosperity: Use this card to manifest a windfall and enjoy the stability created from it. Employ this card to reach finances that fit your version of a comfortable life.

Protection: Use this card to protect your way of life. This safeguards against sudden reversals of fortune.

Love: Use this card to "treat yo' self" to some financial and emotional self-care. This card is about self-sufficiency and will deepen your confidence in yourself.

Clearing: Clear obstacles to your own self-sufficiency. If your goal is to be completely independent, this card will help you realize your favorite version of you.

Healing: Use this card to heal ego after major missteps or repeated attacks on your confidence.

8 of Pentacles

Use this card if you are looking for a new job. This is the apprentice card, so you will be learning a brand-new skill and be starting at the bottom. It's great for opening doors to a new career you have no experience in.

Prosperity: This card is great for finding a new job, particularly if you have just switched careers or are starting out on the next phase of your life. It is fabulous for finding apprenticeships and internships.

Protection: Use this card to protect your position at work.

Love: Use this card for new love, particularly if you are not experienced in the ways of dating. This will bring a partner that will teach you and you can grow together as a couple.

Clearing: Use this card to clear distractions while you are mastering a skill. When used in the reverse, it will help to clear the distractions of small unrelated detail tasks that misdirect you from the large project.

Healing: Use this card to promote feelings of focus and prevent feelings of frustration at a long-term project or improvement.

7 of Pentacles

This is a card of patience for any situation that is growing and ripening without your control. Use it if you need something to manifest without your constant attention.

Prosperity: This card is great for situations that require long-term growth and patience. Use it for investing in the stock market or other long-term hand-off growth opportunities.

Protection: Use this card to guard against situations that will divert your attention from other areas. Use for spells to protect your long-term investments.

Love: Apply this card to bring patience into a relationship when you are both looking for change, growth, and/or resolution.

Clearing: Use the reverse of this card to identify blocks to long-term growth.

Healing: Use this in long-term healing or spiritual development to sustain the work you have already put in.

6 of Pentacles

Use if you are looking for an investor or grant for your idea. This is a card of charity to bring the scales of wealth and poverty into balance. If you employ this card in your spell, make sure you give to charity to start the magic flowing.

Prosperity: This card invites good investors for your projects and business. Don't forget to "pay it forward" after the spell is complete, or your good fortune may go away just as quickly.

Protection: Use this card to protect those you wish to shelter as an act of charity.

Love: Use this card to invite unsolicited love and generosity in your relationships as well as give feelings of love.

Clearing: Use the reverse of this card to identify and clear debts.

Healing: Use this card to heal from the trauma of poverty. Do not be afraid if monetary and emotional offerings and assistance come your way.

5 of Pentacles

This card represents financial loss and an impoverished attitude. Use it in the reversed position to help you rediscover your spiritual wealth, thus bringing new courage, stamina, and ideas to solve your situation. You can also use this card in the beginning of a spell to represent moving from poverty into something better.

Prosperity: Use this card in the reverse to reverse financial loss.

Protection: Use this card to represent a future you wish to protect against.

Love: Use this card in the reverse to counteract long periods without external or self-love and invite prosperous love.

Clearing: Use this card to clear situations and people that continue to keep you in a state of lack in any areas.

Healing: Use this card in directional healing to symbolize moving from poverty or a negative situation toward a positive situation.

4 of Pentacles

This is the miser card, representing a stagnant attitude about money and work and an unwillingness to invest in your future. In the reversed position, it means loss of material things or opportunities. Use it in a spell to represent your struggle and cross it with a card that brings solutions.

Prosperity: Use this card if you have a goal of saving money. This card is best in conjunction with an opportunity card so that you can save toward a goal and not be consumed by your financial obsessions.

Protection: Use this card in an act of self-protection of your current position in life.

Love: Use this card to represent the apprehensions you may be feeling in a relationship to clear and heal them.

Clearing: Use this card to clear situations of monetary hoarding, but be careful to employ this card as the problem card to be crossed with another card to solve the problem.

Healing: Use this card in the reverse to address miserly beliefs about money. In the upright position this card adds control over your healing process around money.

3 of Pentacles

Used to bring more clients and work to you, this card is also helpful in getting a raise and recognition for your skills. If you are looking to increase your willpower in a new health regime, this is the card to use.

Prosperity: Three is a number of motion. Use this card to attract clients to your business; it is particularly good if you are an independent contractor looking for work or a long-term employee looking for a raise or skill recognition.

Protection: Use this card to bring harmony to spirits you work with for protection, particularly if they come in multiples of three. Also use to protect your clients from being stolen from you.

Love: Use this to attract more friends or business connections to help grow professionally and personally.

Clearing: Use this card in reverse to help clear away unhealthy habits that may be holding you back financially.

Healing: Use this card to increase your willpower over your own life, particularly in matters relating to changes in health habits.

2 of Pentacles

Use to help you juggle your finances while you wait for more information or to draw a mentor or guidance.

Prosperity: Use this card to help choose between two or more future opportunities for education or mentorship, for example, grad school, vocational school, or an internship or apprenticeship.

Protection: Use this to protect yourself in a tenuous situation. Apply when living on the edge of poverty and seeking new opportunities.

Love: Use this when relationships seem on the edge of loss to balance work life and personal life.

Clearing: Use this in the reverse to identify and clear overcommitments that do not serve your personal and professional growth.

Healing: Use this card in adaptive healing if you are in a situation that cannot be fully resolved but needs immediate improvement.

SWORDS

The point of the Swords suit is to offer quick and accurate judgment in a situation. This means being swiftly analytical to reach a decision and clarity for a question. The suit is great for general communication and fact-finding. These cards can be fast-acting, but also harsh in their outcomes as they do not adjust facts for emotional reaction. Like the saying goes: "Be careful what you ask for because you just might get it."

Ace of Swords

Use this to overcome creative blocks, inspire new ideas, and communicate in a productive way. This is also a card to dispel evil and negativity.

Prosperity: This card is used to inspire creative thinking and creative communication.
Protection: Use this card in protection spells to think of clever or new methods of protection and adapt to threats.
Love: Use this card to promote creative communication in a relationship.
Clearing: Use this card to clear creative blocks that may be stopping inspiration.
Healing: Use this card to dispel general negativity and evil.

King of Swords

This card represents someone who is quick to judge in his own kingdom. This man is a convincing and inspirational speaker. He is most likely a lawyer, politician, or someone who has to constantly weigh his words. His ideals will always come first, above family and friends. This is a card used to promote brainstorming to look for new ideas. It can also be used to attract legal counsel that will help your case.

Prosperity: This card passes judgment over a large and complex situation. Use it in the communication of your business. Particularly good for those in blue-collar work and those who work with masculine energies.
Protection: Use this card in legal cases to draft the best response or find a competent lawyer.
Love: Use this card to persuade others in your relationships to your point of view and for a calculated edge to business relationships in particular.
Clearing: Use this card in the reverse to add a quiet power to a clearing that needs to be discreet.
Healing: Use this card in the reverse to unlock and use your inner truth.

Queen of Swords

Represents a woman who is a wealth of knowledge and has the intelligence to back it up. She can be a bit aloof and rely on facts only. This card can also mean a completion of a project that communicates new ideas such as a debate, a true story, or developing a speech.

Prosperity: This card is good for researchers, particularly those who are looking into better systems to grow wealth and personally defined prosperity.

Protection: This card is great to use in protective situations that require you to present facts in your defense and deliver arguments against another.

Love: Use this card in situations where you feel another is hiding facts or the truth from you. Be careful, though, because this card will find the facts, but it's up to you what you do with the information.

Clearing: Use this card in the reverse to clear situations that will not respond to logic. As much as we may ask for energy to leave nicely, sometimes a situation only responds to an unemotional bitch.

Healing: Use this card in the upright position to gain control over out-of-control emotions.

Knight of Swords

A talkative young man who cannot stop until he has imposed his opinion on all who are accessible to him. This person is also a gossip and will spread rumors. On the flip side, he will fight to the death for something about which he feels passionate. For travel, it represents travel by air. Use this card for safe travel, in the reversed position to stop gossip, and to get attention for your idea or creation.

Prosperity: Use this card to communicate your ideas and opinions to a large group of people and drive success.

Protection: Use this card to protect you in travel.

Love: Use this card to promote ambition in a relationship. While other cards have been used to answer questions about the next level in a relationship, this card will give you the ambition to grow together and accomplish mutual goals.

Clearing: Use this to quickly and completely empty a space. Best used for surface-level clearings or small to medium-size areas.

Healing: Use this card to heal from burnout, especially after a long semester or leaving a taxing job.

Page of Swords

This card represents an inquisitive child who is always talking and is a know-it-all. This child is quick-witted and solves puzzles easily. As a messenger card, it represents a message that solves a problem or brings a new idea. This is also the card of gossip or, when reversed, to stop gossip.

Prosperity: This is a card of informed exploration. Using your knowledge to explore new paths forward toward prosperity.

Protection: Use this card to protect against idleness and gossip.

Love: Use this to better communicate between yourself and your partner. This card functions especially well during periods of exploration within your relationship. Use this card to clear idle chatter that may be left from a difficult relationship separation.

Clearing: Use this card to clear writer's block.

Healing: Use this card to heal from the destruction of your confidence when gossip has damaged it.

10 of Swords

This is a card that confirms that, indeed, everything that could go wrong did go wrong. It also means the worst is over. If used in a spell, allow it to represent your current condition and cross it with a card that brings courage, healing, and strength to get back up again.

Prosperity: There are some disasters that can be prevented or stopped; use this card to wrap up the end of a financial disaster and stop it from bleeding over into the future.

Protection: Use this card to represent all that has gone wrong and surround it with cards of protection, crossing the top with a card of your leading deities or energy source.

Love: Use this card in communication spells to represent conflict in your relationship and cross it with cards that will heal that rift.

Clearing: Use this card to identify the target of your clearing.

Healing: Use this card in the reverse to aid in recovery from a disaster.

9 of Swords

This is the nightmare card, representing feeling overwhelmed by our own problems. If this is your situation, use the card in the reversed position and surrounded by supportive cards to help you heal your mind and unravel your issues one at a time in a way you can handle.

Prosperity: Use this card to represent your professional doubts and pair it with inspiration and problem-solving cards to change your situation.

Protection: Use this card with a strength card to protect against manifesting nightmares.

Love: Use this card to address anxiety and deep-seated fears in a relationship with a spouse or lover.

Clearing: Use this card to clear your mind of the self-doubt represented by nightmares.

Healing: This is another card you can use to represent yourself with additional cards to aid in healing the nightmare you may be escaping.

8 of Swords

This is a card of imprisonment that is caused by your own fears and lack of courage. If this is your situation, use the card in its reversed position to help free you from this self-entrapment.

Prosperity: This is the card of a victim mentality and represents the lies we tell ourselves about our own actions. Use this card in the reverse to dispel your inner saboteur.

Protection: Use this card to protect against your own self-reducing and any self-harming thoughts. It is great to use when attending intensive therapy or working with a healing practitioner and developing new coping mechanisms to protect yourself.

Love: Use this card with a friend to identify their internal saboteur. It is great for exploring a different perspective. Use it in the reversed position to break out of an abusive relationship that has destroyed your self-worth.

Clearing: Use this card to clear negative thoughts of self-harm and inadequacy.

Healing: Use this card to identify negative thoughts that entrap us and with a healer to move beyond them.

7 of Swords

This is the card of betrayal and theft and implies that someone is stealing from you. Use this card in a spell that reveals a betrayal or to get stolen goods returned to you.

Prosperity: Use this card to protect against professional backstabbing and emotional manipulation.

Protection: Use this card to protect against future attacks from people in your inner circle.

Love: Use this with a friend you suspect of betraying you to reveal the negative actions done against you.

Clearing: Use this card in the reverse to clear feelings of imposter syndrome or those of being an outsider.

Healing: Use this card to find lost property as a victim of theft or fraud.

6 of Swords

This represents a trip by boat. This trip can be to get away from troubles and sorrow, but it can also mean a mental journey to new solutions. You may get assistance with finding your solution from research with the written word.

Prosperity: Use this card when researching a problem. Great for online and archival research.

Protection: Use this card to provide protection abroad, for travel by boat, and to safeguard your mental health and emotions. It is especially good if you are moving into a new and unknown situation.

Love: Use this card with family members to transition into a new stage of growth, whether moving from teenage years into adulthood or moving out for the first time. Use this card to ease your transition into the future.

Clearing: Use this card in the reverse to finish and clear unfinished tasks.

Healing: Here it works to release yourself from emotional baggage.

5 of Swords

This card represents a situation or argument that cannot be won. This can also indicate a failure, a defeat, or an unfair situation. Use it to represent the situation and then cross it with a card that brings a solution.

Prosperity: Use this card in the reverse to reconnect with your business systems and goals.

Protection: Use this card in the reverse to reconcile with your enemies, turning them from problems to allies.

Love: This card predicts conflict and winning an argument above all else. As it is a prediction of stubbornness in a relationship, use this card in reverse to represent an argument and

move it forward toward a mutually beneficial solution and reconciliation.

Clearing: Use this card to represent old disagreements that are still hanging around, and pair it with a card for clearing.

Healing: Use this card to represent your inner conflict with the healing and spiritual development you are working toward. Pair with the Temperance card to bring everything into alignment.

4 of Swords

This is the card of rest after a great stress or illness. In a spell, use this card to cross out and bring relief to a stressful situation.

Prosperity: Use this card to calm a storm at work.

Protection: During long projects use this card in the reverse to protect against burnout and recognize when it's time for a rest.

Love: Use this card to rest your relationships after a traumatic or sudden ending.

Clearing: Use this card to clear situations that will not let you rest when you may need it most.

Healing: Use this to start personal healing from burnout or a long illness. It helps to bring on a meditative relaxation.

3 of Swords

This is the card of heartbreak and unpopular truths being revealed. Use this card if you want the truth of an emotional situation. Another suggested use in a spell is to represent a problem that is crossed with a card that brings solutions.

Prosperity: Use this card to find truths at work. It functions great when crossed with a card that works on finding solutions.

Protection: Use this card to protect against emotional pain and trauma.

Love: Use this card in the upright position to find out truths—often unpleasant ones—about your romantic partner and their emotions. Use this wisely as these truths can likely lead to a breakup.

Clearing: Use this card to clear emotional pain and trauma.

Healing: Use this card in the reverse to release pain.

2 of Swords

This card represents compromise and balance. Use it in spells that need emotional balance and quick, clear decisions.

Prosperity: Employ this card when choosing between two options that will affect your future emotional state.

Protection: Use this card in the reverse to guard against information overload and be able to sort through relevant information.

Love: Use this card when deciding whether or not to continue a relationship with a partner, family, or friends.

Clearing: Clear things that cause your emotions to become unbalanced.

Healing: Use this card to relearn and heal from uncompromising situations within yourself.

WANDS

The Wands are connected with new opportunities. They can often be used with Swords to provide a new path forward out of conflict.

Healing: Use this card in healing, especially if you are working on healing another and need an additional energetic boost.

Ace of Wands

This card represents a new passion or spiritual calling. Use it to power up any situation and give it a new dose of enthusiasm.

Prosperity: Use this card to draw or embrace new opportunities in your professional life or to provide energy to start along a new path.

Protection: Use this card to provide energy to your guides for your general protection.

Love: Use this card to rekindle passions. It is good for romantic partners and professional partners stalled on a project.

Clearing: Use this card to charge your clearing spells with a little extra juice.

King of Wands

This card represents a powerful man who is a true philosopher. He is a very charismatic person who can preach with the best of them. His power radiates from him, and he can be seen as a motivational speaker that moves the crowd to tears and inspires them to change. Use this card in a new-job spell to wow your potential employers. It can also be used for spells to increase your male magnetism or when you need to shore up your position of leadership.

Prosperity: Use this card in a new-job spell to wow your future employers or clients.

Protection: Use this card to protect your position as a leader in a group.

Love: This card works best for those who use male energies in attraction spells.

Clearing: Use this card in the reverse to clear hasty actions and chauvinism.

Healing: Use this card to heal your leadership instincts.

Queen of Wands

This card represents a very charismatic woman who lights up a room when she enters. She is passionate and can be a real fireball; people are very drawn to her. This card can be used in a spell to develop a project that involves travel or a new career. This is also a good card to use in love spells to increase your female magnetism or when you want a boost to your fame.

Prosperity: Use this card to attract competent partners on a new project or a job that involves travel.

Protection: Use this card to protect your strength and self-confidence, especially if you practice servant leadership.

Love: This card is best used by those who work with female energies in attraction spells and popularity spells.

Clearing: Use this card in a clearing spell to persuade rather than boot undesired traits, situations, or people.

Healing: Use this toward the end of a healing journey to reestablish your self-confidence.

Knight of Wands

This card represents a young adult who is very charismatic, almost a party boy. He is popular and does not like to be limited in his ability to travel. Use this card in a spell to manifest a vacation or to steadily increase your fame. Use this card in a spell where you are bucking for a promotion. It can also be used in spells to find a new home and location.

Prosperity: Use this card at work to help your PTO requests or find the backup you need to take a vacation.

Protection: Use this card to ensure your self-care.

Love: Use this card to go on an adventure in your relationship—moving forward with information but taking a great leap of faith together!

Clearing: Use the reverse of this card to clear unnecessary delays in a project.

Healing: Use this card to help find new lodging, especially if you are leaving a traumatic situation.

Page of Wands

This card represents an energetic, creative youth that is filled with ideals about the world. There is a wealth of ideas flowing from this page who is free of the disappointment of failure and the saltiness of adulthood. Use this card to get your ideas flowing freely.

Prosperity: Use this card in the upright position to inspire new thoughts and ideas in a project. Apply it to get a promotion at work. It's great to pair with the Page of Swords card to find solutions to new and unusual problems.

Protection: Use this card in the reverse to tap in to your spiritual leanings and work with or connect to new guides in your protection.

Love: Use this card in discovery, especially to find a new friend group with similar interests.

Clearing: Use this card in reverse at the beginning of a healing spell to redirect and focus your energy on a clearing.

Healing: Use this card to heal your free spirit.

10 of Wands

In a spell, use this card in the reversed position if you are feeling overloaded and need some assistance. This is a wonderful lesson in trying to control too much.

Prosperity: Use this card in the reversed position to get help at work and better spread the load among unhelpful coworkers.
Protection: Use this at the end of lengthy protection processes or for complex protection spells to mark their completion.
Love: Use this card when you need assistance from your romantic partner in your personal life.
Clearing: Use this card in the reversed position to clear and delegate work that is overloading you.
Healing: The healing with this card comes in a release and letting yourself not do it all.

9 of Wands

This card shows you that you are almost to your goal and just need the strength to take the final steps. Use this card in a spell to represent what you are currently experiencing and cross it with a card that will bring a solution.

Prosperity: Use this as a solution card at work, to conquer the final obstacle to finishing a project as a representation of your interests by crossing it with another card to represent the solution.
Protection: Use this card in reverse to call forth your inner reserves to form a protective barrier.
Love: Use this card to set boundaries with a partner or in the final stages of a breakup.
Clearing: Use this card in a clearing spell to close the door behind negative energies removed from your life.
Healing: Use this card in the final stages of healing to reach the finish line.

8 of Wands

This is a card of movement, advancement, and expansion. Use this card in a spell to speed up the positive outcome you desire. It can also represent travel to a faraway place, usually by air.

Prosperity: Use this card in business deals to speed up the process. It is good for legal deals or large sales.
Protection: Use this to protect yourself during long-distance air travel.
Love: Use this spell during matchmaking or speed dating to find your perfect one ASAP.
Clearing: Use this for quick clearings.
Healing: Use this card for quick but short-term healing.

7 of Wands

This card represents the strength to withstand an attack from those who are jealous of you and want to take your power. If you use this card in a spell, surround it with cards that promote strength, courage, and protection.

Prosperity: Use this card to give you strength and courage in a toxic environment.
Protection: Use this card to withstand attacks while you formulate a protection plan.
Love: Use this card to endure toxic relationships that you either cannot or are not ready to sever.
Clearing: Use this card to get you straight in clearing your own realm.
Healing: Use this card to give you courage to face a long healing journey.

6 of Wands

This is the card you would use in a spell to represent victory! This is the recognition and reward for a job well done. This is the culmination of success.

Prosperity: Use this card to represent success in your professional life, whether for a new job, promotion, or finished project.

Protection: Use this in protection to triumph over evil in your life. The best defense sometimes is a good offense.

Love: Use this for goals within a relationship that you are both or all working toward. This can be buying a house with a partner, finishing a project, or finally having that whole family reunion.

Clearing: Use this card to represent a successful clearing. It is great for long-term clearings and physical decluttering.

Healing: Use this card to represent the end of a healing journey. This card will help you manifest your personal rewards at the end of this phase.

5 of Wands

This is a card that represents a power struggle between equals. Use it in the reversed position to bring courage to face this situation, stand out, make a positive statement, and create new opportunities for yourself—and, oh, yeah, create harmony in the workplace.

Prosperity: Use this card to represent harmony in the workplace.

Protection: Use this card in the reverse to represent conflict avoidance in tense situations.

Love: Use this card between friends or partners to represent harmony in the relationship.

Clearing: Use this card to represent a power struggle between you and a particularly difficult block.

Healing: Use this card to identify disharmony in your life to be healed.

4 of Wands

Use this card in your spell to denote stability and reward for your hard work, commitment, and good decisions. This card can also be used to bring about a marriage.

Prosperity: Use this card to win or attract professional awards such as bonuses, raises, honors, and promotions.

Protection: Use this card to bring consistency and predictability.

Love: Use this card to bring stability into your family and personal life.

Clearing: Use this card in a clearing spell to bring it stability and focus as it clears out its target.

Healing: Use this card after healing to manifest a stable situation.

3 of Wands

Use this card in your spell to represent the next step of progress in the situation in which you are invested. It also denotes a partner in business, profitable trade, commerce, and personal pride.

Prosperity: Use this card to figure out the next step in your investment or personal business. Great for business owners that are looking to expand.

Protection: Use this card in the reverse to protect from potential shortsightedness.

Love: Use this when you're ready to expand your romantic relationship, particularly if you are invested for the long term.

Clearing: Use this card in the reverse to clear short-term goals.

Healing: Use this card to heal injuries to your ego, particularly when you are not recognized for your hard work.

2 of Wands

Use this card to help you make a choice, especially when two equally viable options are presented to you. This card will work to ensure that you are making the right one and bring you the courage to do so.

Prosperity: Use this card to choose between two options in your future planning.

Protection: Use this card in the reverse to protect your personal goals while you make decisions about your growth.
Love: Use this card after speed dating to clear your mind and make a romantic choice.
Clearing: Use this card in the reverse to ensure that your clearing aligns with your personal goals.
Healing: Use this card in the reverse to address inner conflict and personally inflicted emotional deficits.

CUPS

Cups are particularly good for building and maintaining relationships of all types—family, friend, and partner. They represent the primal intuition that can rule our habits and reactions to others and our environment.

Ace of Cups

Use this card in a spell to represent a new love in your life.

Prosperity: Use this card to spark new creativity and imagination.
Protection: Use this card in the reverse to boost your intuition in new situations.
Love: Use this card to represent a new love in your life, and cross it with other cards to attract or solidify this new love.
Clearing: Use this card in the reverse to clear repressed emotions about a targeted situation.
Healing: Use this card in the reverse to heal your self-love.

King of Cups

This card represents a kind gentleman who is dedicated to his family and children. He is emotionally stable, and his waters run deep. He will do just about anything to protect his people. Use this card in a spell to promote a marriage proposal or to be asked on a date.

Prosperity: Use this card in business deals that need an even hand and diplomacy to let your ideas come across.
Protection: Use this card for family protection, particularly if you work in male energies.
Love: Use this card to bring emotional stability to your relationships.
Clearing: Use this card in reverse to clear feelings and situations that may be emotionally manipulating you.
Healing: Use this card to promote compassion for your own healing or particularly if you are helping another.

Queen of Cups

This card represents a woman who is a healer and/or psychic. She is very empathic and can help with any emotional situation. She may be shy but is the first to be supportive and nurturing. Use this card to represent your growing interest in a romantic situation. You can also use it in spells to deepen your psychic connections.

Prosperity: This card is best for those who work with female energies to tap into psychic powers for your prosperity.
Protection: Use this card to protect yourself as you work in healing energies or to perform spells for others.
Love: Use this card to take a new love from the "talking phase" to the "relationship phase"—in spells, it will act to make your Facebook relationship status official!
Clearing: Use this to enhance your psychic ability when searching out energetic and spiritual blocks.
Healing: This is a great card for healers who work in female energies to heal themselves and others.

Knight of Cups

This card represents a young adult who is all about love and romance, a Romeo in the fullest sense of the word. He is very deep emotionally and can be moody. Use this card in a spell to represent the transition of a relationship from dating to a more serious partnership.

Prosperity: Use this card in the reverse with protection cards to limit unrealistic expectations when working on a work project.
Protection: Use this card to bring someone that will help protect your heart and emotions in a stressful situation.
Love: This card is a good conduit to the next step in your relationship. It is particularly good for young adults and those who have had no or few partners.
Clearing: This card is good to help clear your doubts about being lovable.
Healing: This card will help heal your issues around being attractive and desirable.

Page of Cups

A very artistic and creative child is represented by this card. This child is recognized as a dreamer and very sensitive. This card can also be used to represent a message of love and romance coming your way.

Prosperity: This card is best utilized by artists who want to sell their work and remain inspired.
Protection: Use this card to protect your sensitive side and keep it from becoming jaded.
Love: This card is a messenger of love—someone is thinking about you! Take your shot.
Clearing: Use this to clear creative blocks and emotional immaturity.
Healing: Use this in spells for the healing of children or your inner child. Cross with the Sun card to fully heal innocent youth.

10 of Cups

Use this card in your spell for family bliss. This is the card for a balanced, secure home with lasting happiness.

Prosperity: Use this card in reverse when you are ready to realign your business practices with harmony and respect.
Protection: Use this card to symbolize yourself and your family as the objects to be protected, and cross with other cards.
Love: Use this for contentment and harmony within the family.
Clearing: Use this card in the reverse to identify disharmony in a family and balance it.
Healing: Use this card in spells to heal struggling relationships.

9 of Cups

This card is the wish-fulfillment card. Use it in a spell just for that. What you wish for, you will get! You will live large, have the best, and be willing to share with friends.

Prosperity: Use this card at work to fulfill wishes, particularly those with a slim chance of realization.
Protection: Use this card in the reverse to protect your inner peace.
Love: Use this card to fulfill a wish in your relationship.
Clearing: Use this card to boost your clearing spells. Make a wish to expedite issues or forever seal them into the past.
Healing: Use this card to add some cosmic will and wish into your healing process, especially if you are helping to heal others.

8 of Cups

This card can be used in a spell to gain the courage needed to make a profound life change that will take you in an unknown direction.

Prosperity: Use this card to gather the courage to start a new business, quit your old job, or start a new career across the country.
Protection: Use this card to gather the courage to start the protection process, particularly against people and situations that stand in the way of you and your romantic interests.
Love: This card is great to gather courage to make a big romantic change. Turn a friend into a partner or ask a partner about marriage.
Clearing: Use this card in the reverse to know when it is time to walk away from a situation.
Healing: Use this card in the upright position with other strength cards to aid in your healing goals.

7 of Cups

This card represents too many choices and having a false and romantic perception of all of them. If this is your situation, use this card in the reversed position to bring clarity to your choices. It will also bring determination, will-power, and the correct decision.

Prosperity: Use this card in the reverse to get rid of too many choices. Cross this with a goals card to focus your decision-making process.
Protection: Use this card to protect and center your personal alignment and values in your decision-making process.
Love: Use this card in reverse to help make choices. It's perfect after a round of dates to decide on the perfect match.
Clearing: Use this card to declutter excess from your life.
Healing: Use this card to heal yourself from illusions of success.

6 of Cups

Use this card in your spell to represent perfect bliss and happiness. This is also a card of innocence and childhood. Possibly use it to bring someone from your past or childhood back into your life.

Prosperity: Use this card to achieve pure joy and wonderment in your professional career.
Protection: Use this card to protect your inner child and sense of wonder.
Love: Use this card to find those from your past, particularly childhood friends or relationships that bring childlike innocence and wonder back into your life.
Clearing: Use this card in the reverse to clear reminders and past issues.
Healing: Use this card in inner child or child healing spells.

5 of Cups

This is a card of sorrow, regret, and despair. Where so much energy is spent on sorrow, you cannot see what you still have. If this card represents your situation, use it in your spell in the reversed position to return hope, love, and courage to your life.

Prosperity: Use this card in the reverse to represent moving beyond setbacks in your professional life.
Protection: Use this card in the reverse to protect against bone-chilling sorrow.
Love: Use this card in reverse to undo feelings of despair and move on from a romantic separation or ending.
Clearing: Use this card in the reverse to banish the situations causing you sorrow.
Healing: Use this card in the reverse to represent your situation and cross it with other cards to represent where you'd like to move forward. Use this card to forgive yourself.

4 of Cups

This is a card that represents dissatisfaction in everything, usually caused by too much stimulation.

Prosperity: Use this card in the reverse to move melancholy and dissatisfaction out of your workspace.
Protection: Use this card to protect your inner peace and mindfulness.
Love: Use this card in reverse to get rid of over-stimulating factors to your relationship.
Clearing: Use this card to clear distraction from a large and important task.
Healing: Use this card in reverse to heal from long periods of unwanted self-isolation.

3 of Cups

This card represents an overflowing of love—lots and lots of love. It can also be used for overall general good fortune.

Prosperity: Use this card to bring joy into your professional life.
Protection: Use this card in a protection spell for others, particularly a long-term friend.
Love: Use this card to provide an abundance of love in a relationship.
Clearing: Use this to focus a friendship clearing to dispel feelings and people that don't provide the desired collaborations.
Healing: This card in the reverse is particularly helpful for currently sober people to heal from the chemical abuse of their past.

2 of Cups

In a spell, this card would represent a budding relationship that is in the first stages of romance. It can also represent finding your soul mate.

Prosperity: This is another card for choosing; however, its best effects are in matters of the heart. Just this author's advice, but avoid office romances if you aren't ready to see your spouse every day.
Protection: Use this card to represent the love you would like to protect.
Love: Use this at the beginning of a relationship to build a strong soul mate bond.
Clearing: Use this card to clear the path to a new relationship.
Healing: Use this card in the reverse to represent a breakup with your partner that you are ready to move beyond.

SYMBOLS INDEX

Based in the art of tea reading, the following symbols and their potential meanings are a starting point for your wax interpretations. Thanks to Heatherleigh Navarre of the Boston Tea Room in Ferndale, Michigan, for her guidance in creating this list. Heatherleigh is a third-generation tea leaf reader, powerful witch, and an amazing friend.

Arrow: Direction, focus

Bird: Vision, clarity

Book: Imagination, tradition

Boot: Travel, work, industry

Bundle: Search for truth

Cat: Impetuousness, curiosity

Chair: Marriage, stagnation

Circles: Great success

Coins: Material security

Cross: Religious quest

Crown: Leadership, ego

Dog: Loyalty, dependability

Eye: Soul, introspection

Feather: Flight, independence, wanderlust

Flame: Creativity, art

Hand: Helpmate, relationship

Heart: Love, emotion, partnership

Key: Knowledge, education, opportunity

Leaf: Fertility, nature, energy

Letters: References to the names of friends or relatives

Moon: Denial, female intuition

Numbers: Indicators of spans of time, such as months or years

Owl: Wisdom, isolation, nocturnal

Shovel: Manual labor, hidden depths

Squares: The need for caution

Star: Spirituality, popularity

Sun: Enlightenment, happiness, children

Tree: Family, stability

Triangles: Good karma

Vase: Material concerns

MAGIC 5 INDEX OF INGREDIENTS

With all the magic possibilities you have been inspired to create throughout the course of *The Big Book of Candle Magic,* it can quickly get overwhelming to figure out where to start. Use this index of ingredients as a quick *start* guide to building a spell in one of the Magic 5 categories, and then let your intuition guide you to happy little accidents that make the spell perfect for your need.

PROSPERITY/MONEY DRAW/MATERIAL GAIN/SUCCESS MAGIC

Candle Type
Blessed candles specific to your purpose
Any votive, taper, chime, tealight, seven-day, or
    pillar candle in the appropriate color
Seven-knob candle
Cat figure candle
Devil figure candle
Pyramid figure candle

Phase of the Moon
New
Waxing
Full

Moon Sign
Aries
Taurus
Leo
Virgo
Capricorn
Aquarius

Color
Aqua/Teal
Brown
Gold
Green
Orange
Purple
Red
Yellow

Herbs/Oils
Allspice
Arnica
Basil
Bay Leaves
Bergamot
Catnip
Cedar
Chamomile
Cinnamon
Citrus (all)

Clove
Coriander
Cumin
Dandelion
Dates and Figs
Dill Weed
Dragon's Blood
Evergreen
Five Finger Grass
Ginger
Honeysuckle
Irish Moss
Lemon Balm
Lemongrass
Mustard Seeds
Myrrh
Nutmeg
Oakmoss
Orange Blossom (Neroli)
Parsley
Patchouli
Pennyroyal
Poppy
Sage
Sassafras
Turmeric
Uva-ursi

Stone
Amber
Aventurine
Bloodstone
Calcite (all colors)
Carnelian
Citrine
Jade

Lodestone (Magnetite)
Quartz Crystal
Selenite
Sunstone
Turquoise

Tarot Cards
Magician
Emperor
Wheel of Fortune
Devil
Sun
Pentacles

Curio
Black Cat Hair
Crossroad
Crown
Dice
Flowers
High John the Conqueror Root
Horseshoe
Lodestone
Magnetic Sand
Money
Red Flannel
Shells

Symbol
Circle
Coins
Crown
Key
Leaf
Triangles
Vase

PROTECTION/SAFETY MAGIC

Candle Type
Blessed candles specific to your purpose
Any votive, taper, chime, tealight, seven-day, or
    pillar candle in the appropriate color
Cat figure candle
Cross figure candle

Phase of the Moon
New
Waxing
Full

Moon Sign
Aries
Taurus
Libra
Scorpio
Capricorn

Color
Black
Brown
Silver
White

Herbs/Oils
Agrimony
Angelica
Anise
Bay Leaves
Blessed Thistle
Cardamom
Cayenne, Chili Pepper, Paprika
Cedar
Comfrey
Cypress
Dill Weed
Dragon's Blood
Eucalyptus
Evergreen
Fennel
Frankincense
Garlic
Geranium
Ginger
Juniper
Mustard Seeds
Myrrh
Nettles
Nightshade(s)
Parsley
Pennyroyal
Peppercorn
Rose
Rosemary
Rowan
Rue
Saffron/Safflower
Sandalwood
Tarragon
Turmeric

Stone
Amazonite
Amber
Amethyst
Aquamarine
Bloodstone
Carnelian
Emerald
Fluorite
Garnet
Hematite
Jade
Jasper
Jet
Labradorite
Lapis
Lodestone (Magnetite)
Obsidian, Black

Petrified Wood
Quartz Crystal
Selenite
Snowflake Obsidian
Tourmaline, Black
Turquoise

Tarot Cards
Magician
High Priestess
Strength
Hermit
Justice
Moon
Swords

Curio
Black Cat Hair

Cascarilla
Crossroads
Horseshoe
Money
Railroad Spike
Red Flannel
Salt
Scissors
Skeleton Key
Tobacco

Symbol
Cross
Dog
Eye
Tree
Triangles

LOVE/RELATIONSHIP/COMMUNICATION MAGIC

Candle Type
Blessed candles specific to your purpose
Any votive, taper, chime, tealight, seven-day, or
    pillar candle in the appropriate color
Devil figure candle
Genitalia figure candle
Human figure candle
Lovers figure candle
Marriage figure candle

Phase of the Moon
New
Waxing
Full

Moon Sign
Gemini
Cancer
Leo
Libra

Color
Aqua/Teal
Green
Orange
Pink
Red

Herbs/Oils
Allspice
Althea
Angelica
Anise
Balsam of Peru
Basil
Catnip
Cinnamon
Clove
Coriander
Damiana
Dates and Figs

Ginger
Honeysuckle
Jasmine
Lavender
Marjoram
Mint (all)
Orange Blossom (Neroli)
Patchouli
Peony
Poppy
Rose
Savory
Thyme
Vanilla
Ylang-Ylang

Stone
Agate (all types)
Amethyst
Carnelian
Emerald
Garnet
Lodestone (Magnetite)
Moonstone
Opal
Quartz Crystal
Rose Quartz

Selenite
Turquoise

Tarot Cards
High Priestess
Empress
Hierophant
Lovers
Cups

Curio
Black Cat Hair
Crossroads
Feather
Flowers
High John the Conqueror Root
Lodestone
Red Flannel
Shells
Skull

Symbol
Arrow
Chair
Leaf
Sun
Tree

CLEARING/OPENING MAGIC

Candle Type
Blessed candles specific to your purpose
Any votive, taper, chime, tealight, seven-day, or
    pillar candle in the appropriate color
Devil figure candle

Phase of the Moon
Full
Waning

Moon Sign
Gemini
Virgo
Scorpio
Sagittarius
Capricorn
Aquarius
Pisces

Color
Aqua/Teal

Black
Blue
Purple
Silver
White

Herbs/Oils
Agrimony
Aloe
Althea
Bay Leaves
Blessed Thistle
Cayenne, Chili Pepper, Paprika
Celery Seed
Chamomile
Copal
Cypress
Dandelion
Eucalyptus
Frankincense
Geranium
Hyssop
Juniper
Lemon Balm
Lemongrass
Nettles
Nightshade(s)
Orange Blossom (Neroli)
Pennyroyal
Peony
Peppercorn
Rosemary
Sage
Saint-John's-Wort
Uva-ursi
Valerian
Vervain

Stone
Amazonite
Amethyst
Aquamarine
Aventurine

Calcite (all colors)
Fluorite
Hematite
Jet
Lapis
Lepidolite
Lodestone (Magnetite)
Moonstone
Obsidian, Black
Quartz Crystal
Selenite
Sodalite
Tourmaline, Black
Turquoise

Tarot Cards
Fool
Chariot
Hanged Man
Death
Tower
Moon
Sun
Judgement
Wands

Curio
Cascarilla
Crossroads
Feather
Flowers
Railroad Spike
Red Flannel
Salt
Scissors
Shells
Skeleton Key
Tobacco

Symbol
Bird
Feather
Moon

THE BIG BOOK OF CANDLE MAGIC

HEALING/BALANCING MAGIC

Candle Type
Blessed candles specific to your purpose
Any votive, taper, chime, tealight, seven-day, or
     pillar candle in the appropriate color
Human figure candle
Skull figure candle

Phase of the Moon
Full
Waning

Moon Sign
Aries
Taurus
Cancer
Virgo
Scorpio
Sagittarius

Color
Aqua/Teal
Black
Blue
Brown
Gold
Green
Orange
Pink
Purple
Silver
White

Herbs/Oils
Allspice
Aloe
Althea
Angelica
Anise
Balsam of Peru
Basil
Bergamot
Cardamom
Catnip
Celery Seed
Citrus (all)
Comfrey
Copal
Dragon's Blood
Evergreen
Fennel
Frankincense
Ginger
Jasmine
Mugwort
Mustard Seeds
Myrrh
Nutmeg
Patchouli
Poppy
Rose
Saffron/Safflower
Saint-John's-Wort
Sandalwood
Savory
Thyme
Turmeric
Uva-ursi
Valerian
Wormwood
Yarrow

Stone
Agate (all types)
Amazonite
Amber
Amethyst
Aquamarine
Aventurine
Bloodstone
Calcite (all colors)

Carnelian
Emerald
Fluorite
Jade
Jasper
Jet
Labradorite
Lapis
Lepidolite
Moonstone
Obsidian, Black
Opal
Petrified Wood
Quartz Crystal
Rose Quartz
Selenite
Serpentine
Sodalite
Sunstone
Tigereye
Turquoise

Tarot Cards
High Priestess
Empress
Strength

Temperance
Star
Sun
World
Wands

Curio
Crossroads
Crown
Feather
Flowers
High John the Conqueror Root
Red Flannel
Shells
Skeleton Key
Skull
Tobacco

Symbol
Arrow
Book
Eye
Leaf
Sun
Triangles

BOTANICAL
CLASSIFICATION INDEX

Agrimony (*Agrimonia eupatoria*)

Allspice (*Pimenta dioica*)

Aloe (*Aloe ferox*)

Althea Root (Marshmallow) (*Althaea officinalis*)

Angelica (*Angelica archangelica*)

Anise (*Pimpinella anisum*)

Arnica (*Arnica montana*)

Balsam of Peru (*Myroxylon balsamum*)

Basil (*Ocimum basilicum*)

Bay Leaves (*Laurus nobilis*)

Bergamot (*Citrus bergamia*)

Blessed Thistle (*Cnicus benedictus*)

Cardamom (*Elettaria cardamomum*)

Catnip (*Nepeta cataria*)

Cayenne/Chili Peppers/Paprika (*Capsicum annuum*)

Cedar (*Thuja plicata*)

Celery Seed (*Apium graveolens*)

Chamomile (*Matricaria recutita*)

Cinnamon, Indonesian (*Cinnamomum burmanii*)

Citronella Essential Oil (*Cymbopogon winterianus*)

Citrus Family (*Citrus*)

    Grapefruit (*Citrus paradisi*)

    Lemon (*Citrus limon*)

    Lime (*Citrus aurantifolia*)

    Orange (*Citrus sinensis*)

    Tangerine (*Citrus reticulata*)

Clove (*Syzygium aromaticum*)

Comfrey (*Symphytum officinale*)

Copal (*Protium copal, Bureseru microphylla*)

Coriander (*Coriandrum sativum*)

Cumin (*Cuminum cyminum*)

Cypress (*Cupressus sempervirens*)

Damiana (*Turnera diffusa*)

Dandelion (*Taraxacum officinale*)

Date (*Phoenix dactylifera*)

Dill Weed (*Anethum graveolens*)

Dragon's Blood (*Daemonorops draco*)

Eucalyptus (*Eucalyptus globulus*)

Evergreens (Fir and Pine)

    Fir (*Abies sibirica*)

    Pine (*Pinus sylvestris*)

Fennel (*Foeniculum vulgare var. dulce*)

Figs (*Ficus carica*)

Five Finger Grass (Cinquefoil) (*Potentilla erecta*)

Frankincense (Ethiopia: *Boswellia papyrifera*, India: *Boswellia serrata*)

Garlic (*Allium sativum*)

Geranium (*Pelargonium graveolens*)

Ginger (*Zingiber officinale*)

Honeysuckle (*Lonicera japonica*)

Hyssop (*Hyssopus officinalis*)

Irish Moss (Sea moss) (*Chondrus crispus*)

Jasmine (*Jasminum odoratissimum*)

Juniper (*Juniperus communis*)

Lavender (*Lavandula x intermedia*)

Lemon balm (*Melissa officinalis*)

Lemon grass

    essential (*Cymbopogon flexuosus*)

    herb (*Cymbopogon citratus*)

Marjoram (*Origanum majorana*)
Mints (*Mentha*)
   Peppermint (*Mentha piperita*)
   Spearmint (*Mentha spicata*)
   Wintergreen (*Gaultheria procumbens*)
Mugwort (*Artemisia vulgaris*)
Mustard Seeds
   brown (*Brassica juncea*)
   white (*Sinapis alba*)
Myrrh (*Commiphora molmol*)
Nettles (*Urtica dioica*)
Belladonna (*Atropa belladonna*) nightshade
Nutmeg (*Myristica fragrans*)
Oakmoss (*Evernia prunastri*)
Orange Blossom (Neroli) (*Citrus aurantium*)
Orris Root (Iris) (*Iris x germanica*)
Parsley (*Petroselinum crispum*)
Patchouli (*Pogostemon cablin*)
Pennyroyal (*Mentha pulegium*)
Peony (*Paeonia lactiflora*)
Peppercorn (*Piper nigrum*)
Poppy Seed (*Papaver somniferum*)

Rose (*Rosa centifolia*)
Rosemary (*Rosmarinus officinalis*)
Rowan (*Sorbus aucuparia*)
Rue (*Ruta graveolens*)
Safflower (*Carthamus tinctorius*)
Saffron (*Crocus sativus*)
Sage (*Salvia officinalis*)
Saint-John's-Wort (*Hypericum perforatum*)
Sandalwood (*Santalum album*)
Sassafras (*Sassafras albidum*)
Savory (*Satureja hortensis*)
Star Anise (*Illicium verum*)
Tarragon (*Artemisia dracunculis*)
Turmeric (*Curcuma longa*)
Thyme (*Thymus vulgaris*)
Uva-ursi (*Arctostaphylos uva-ursi*)
Valerian (*Valeriana officinalis*)
Vanilla (*Vanilla planifolia*)
Vervain (*Verbena officinalis*)
Wormwood (*Artemisia absinthium*)
Yarrow (*Achillea millefolium*)
Ylang-Ylang (*Cananga odorata*)

INDEX

THE BIG BOOK OF CANDLE MAGIC

TO OUR READERS